ESSENTIAL WELLNESS

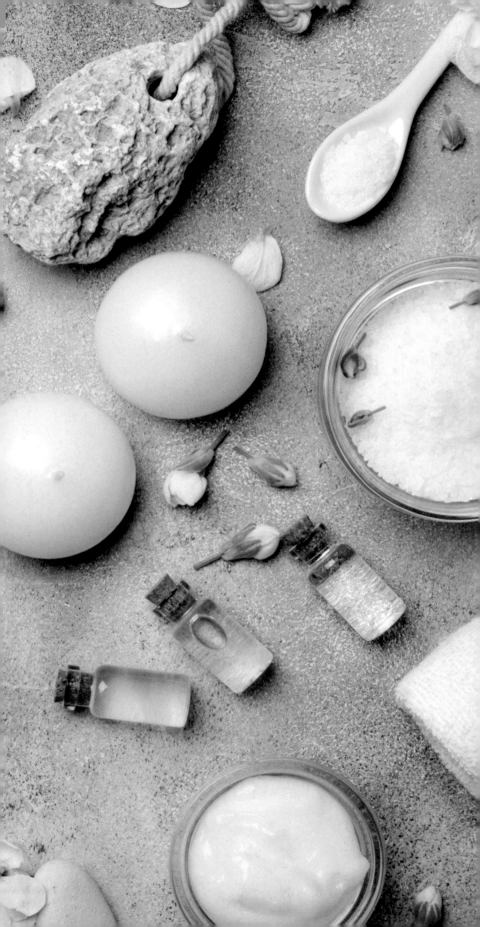

ESSENTIAL WELLNESS

YOGA, MEDITATION, HERBAL REMEDIES, SPA TREATMENTS, MASSAGE, and MORE

Natural solutions for health and well-being

Nancy J. Hajeski

ThunderBay
P·R·E·S·S

San Diego, California

Thunder Bay Press
An imprint of Printers Row Publishing Group
10350 Barnes Canyon Road, Suite 100, San Diego, CA 92121
www.thunderbaybooks.com

Thunder Bay Press
Publisher: Peter Norton
Associate Publisher: Ana Parker
Publishing/Editorial Team: April Farr, Vicki Jaeger, Kelly Larsen, Stephanie Romero, Kathryn C. Dalby, Carrie Davis
Editorial Team: JoAnn Padgett, Melinda Allman
Production Team: Jonathan Lopes, Rusty von Dyl

Produced by Moseley Road Inc., www.moseleyroad.com
President: Sean Moore
Production Director: Adam Moore
Cover Designer: Lisa Purcell
Supplemental Writers: Grace Moore, Finn Moore, Nancy J. Hajeski

Library of Congress Cataloging-in-Publication data is available upon request.

ISBN: 978-1-68412-639-2

Printed in China

23 22 21 20 19   1 2 3 4 5

CONTENTS

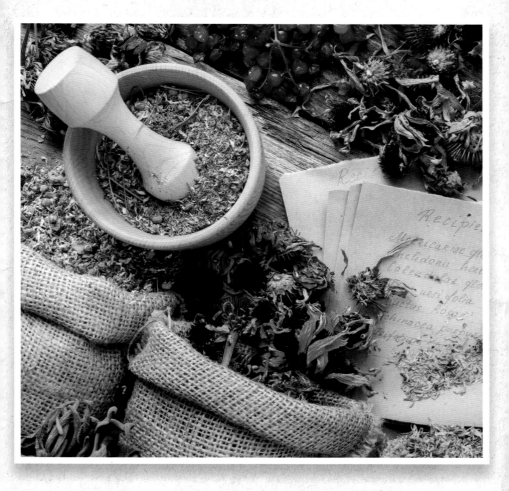

EMBRACING WELLNESS

Today, many people are educating themselves on the benefits of a healthier lifestyle. This new focus may occur as the result of illness, aging, an emotional turning point, or simply a budding desire to do whatever is possible to support overall well being. This book offers guidelines for making the right decisions when it comes to improving how to move, how to breathe, how to take care of yourself, and, ultimately, how to live.

ADVANCING SLOWLY BUT SURELY

The best part of making a conscientious effort to increase levels of wellness in your life is that you can start relatively small—perhaps adding a half hour of exercise to your daily routine and eating a salad once a day—and gradually progress to tackling bigger, more unilateral changes.

A few steps in the right direction can often lead to surprising results, results that encourage you to stay with a program. You don't need to become a yoga master during the first few months you practice the discipline . . . just learning

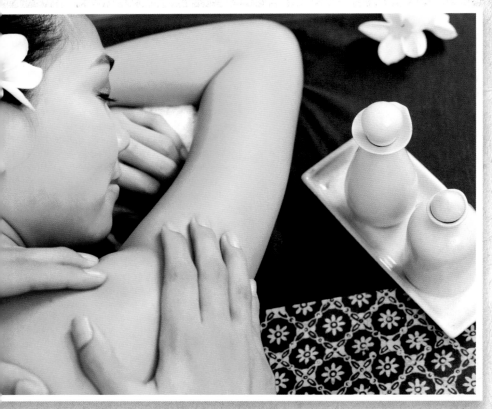

Massage is physically and spiritually soothing (above); meditation space (opposite).

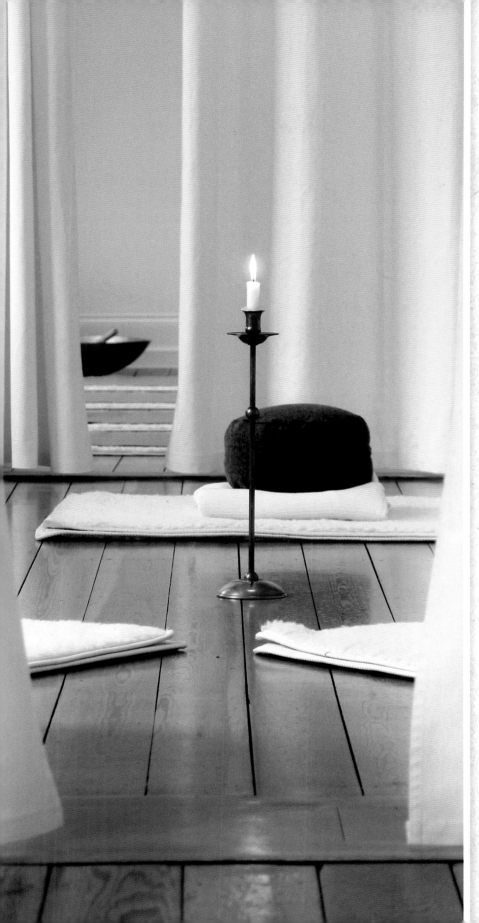

to breathe and focus are already beneficial outcomes. Yet the better you feel, the more likely you are to stick with any new wellness program. The same goes for meditation or massage . . . if you are able to achieve a relaxed state with a relatively quiet mind, you are well on your way to lowering stress. And the more relaxed you feel, the better the chances you will continue to deepen your knowledge of either pursuit.

The point of almost every aspect of wellness is to feel that you are in control of your body and mind and are working toward becoming a better, healthier version of yourself. Whether that involves exercise, meditation, massage, addressing illness with healing herbs and essential oils, enhancing your appearance, establishing a chemical-free home, or preparing nutritious beverages, this book will help you to heighten your levels of understanding . . . and increase the subsequent rewards.

YOGA—MIND AND BODY

Yoga has been offering a range of physical, psychological, and spiritual benefits for thousands of years. Within this book you will learn a number of beginner and intermediate poses—called asanas—that will help relieve tension in your neck, shoulders, back, lower body, and core and will also provide a calming, stress-lowering experience that has few equals.

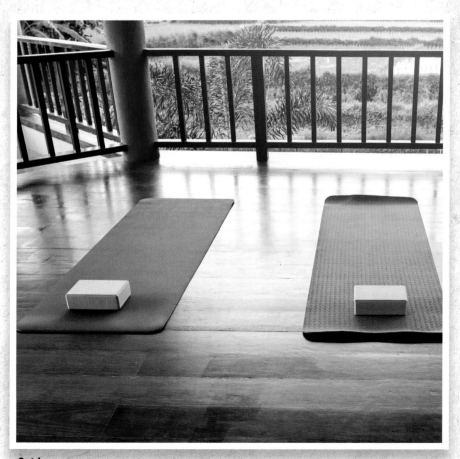

Outdoor yoga space

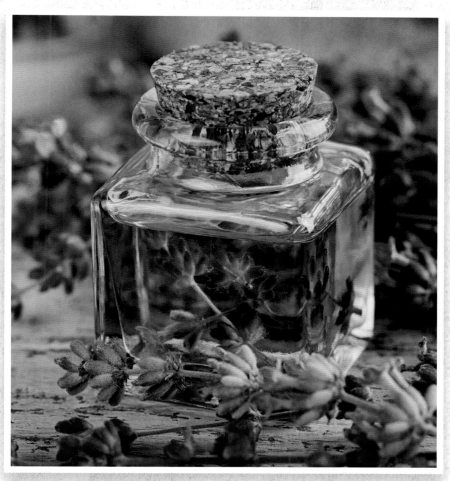

Lavender massage oil

MEDITATION—MIND OVER MATTER

Meditation is an ancient practice that allows people to seek insights and enlightenment by counteracting the demands of daily life and reducing the "chatter" of the over-burdened brain. By looking inward and focusing on rhythmic breathing, you can soon achieve a deeper state of consciousness that will relax your body, refresh your spirit, and renew your mental energies.

HERBAL SOLUTIONS—NATURE'S OWN REMEDIES

Herbal medicines—herbs, spices, and other botanicals—have been used for thousands of years by natural healers, and they continue to offer a wide array of cures, treatments, and aids. Learn which herbs are effective remedies for a variety of ailments, including insomnia, emotional distress, and the side effects of pregnancy.

ESSENTIAL OILS—BREATHE DEEP

First distilled by the ancients, the essential oils of herbs, spices, and other botanicals have recently been rediscovered—and lauded—by the natural health community. When blended with carrier oils, these aromatic, concentrated oils can ease pain, aid breathing, clear foggy thinking, and even enhance libido.

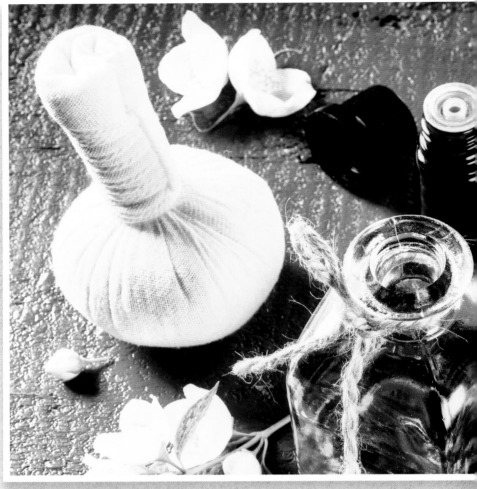

Spa accessories, including essential and massage oils, bath salts, and massage ball

SPA THERAPY—BEAUTIFY AT HOME

What could be more indulgent than providing yourself with customized skin, hair, and nail treatments in your own tranquil home spa? Discover tips for creating a spa-like environment in your own bathroom, as well as recipes for preparing nourishing balms, moisturizers, scrubs, shampoos, conditioners, and bath fizzies from products in your pantry.

MASSAGE—HANDS-ON RELIEF

Whether you desire a "classical" massage or something a bit more rigorous, you'll learn the different modalities available to clients at massage salons, health spas, and physical therapy centers. You can also determine which type of massage meets your needs, understand how to set a fee beforehand, and even figure out how much to tip—or know when not to tip.

THE HEALTHY HOME—ELIMINATE HIDDEN TOXINS

Most households contain five or six commercial cleaners, each with its own list of toxic ingredients. Avoid this daily over exposure to chemicals by replacing those harsh cleaners with safe, effective pantry products.

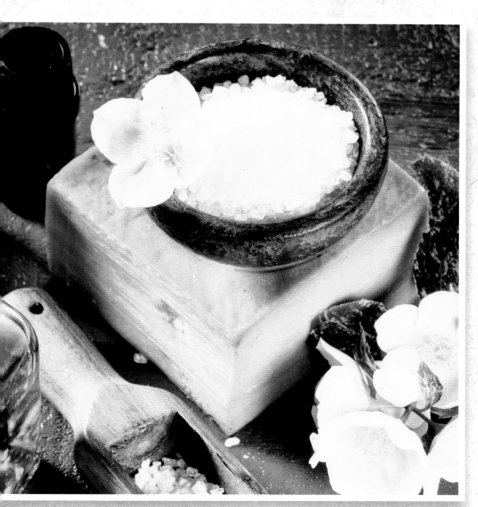

Vinegar, baking soda, lemon juice, and salts can be used to wipe down, spot clean, de-grease, scrub, sanitize, deodorize, and even disinfect counters, sinks, floors, carpets, appliances, and other surfaces in the kitchen and bath and around the house.

TEAS, TONICS, AND SMOOTHIES—DRINK UP!

We all know how important hydration is for keeping the body in good health. Here you will find a whole chapter of drinks made with herbs and spices that add nutritional benefits to the concept of hydration. Try these recipes for hot or cold teas, time-tested health tonics, antioxidant smoothies, and tasty smoothie bowls.

Whatever area or areas you choose to focus on as you begin your "wellness makeover"—and this guidebook gives you plenty of physical and psychological options— remember that lifestyle changes often take time to set seed and take root. Yet the lasting rewards eventually outweigh any sense of discouragement or frustration you may feel at first. Stick with your new program, and you will soon begin to experience the uplifting effects of improved health and emotional well being that will inspire you to carry on.

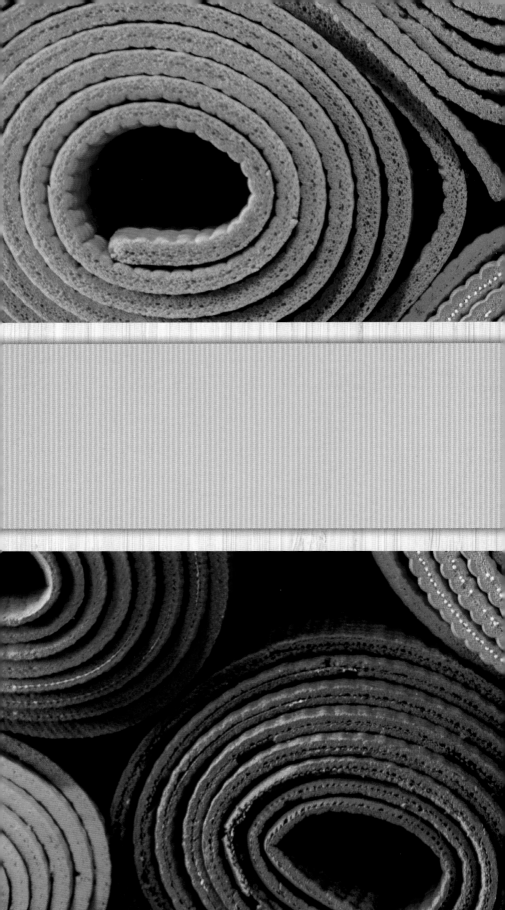

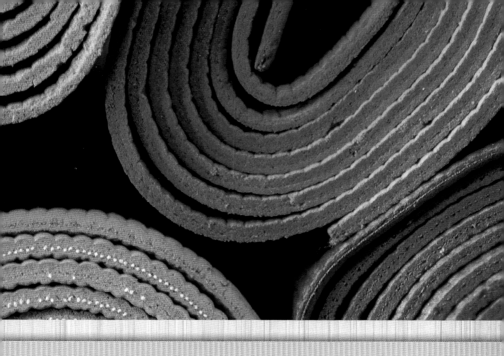

CHAPTER 1
THE MANY BENEFITS OF YOGA

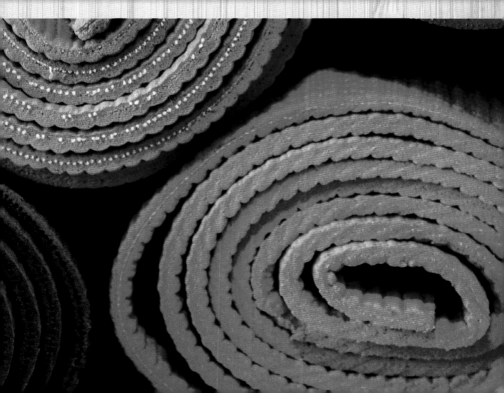

THE MANY BENEFITS OF YOGA

Yoga became increasingly popular with health-conscious individuals during the latter part of the twentieth century and has continued its rise into the new millennium. What was once the pursuit of American eccentrics and "health nuts" is now an accepted mainstream form of exercise that strengthens, stretches, and tones the body, improves circulation, and calms the mind and spirit.

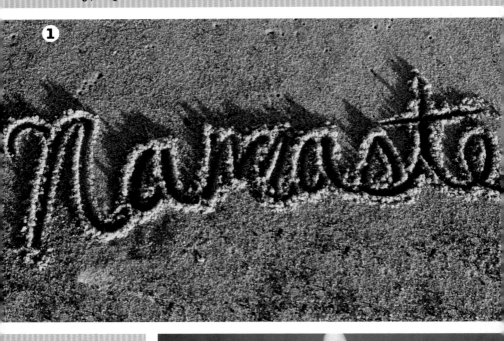

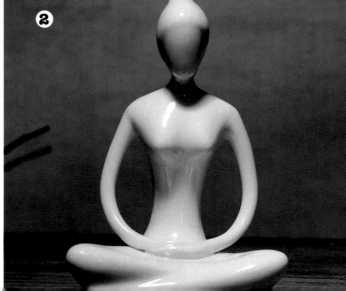

1 Namaste is a form of greeting in Hindu custom
2 Modern yoga lady
3 Yoga studio
4 Setting the mood
5 Yogi seated in a garden
6 Triangle pose

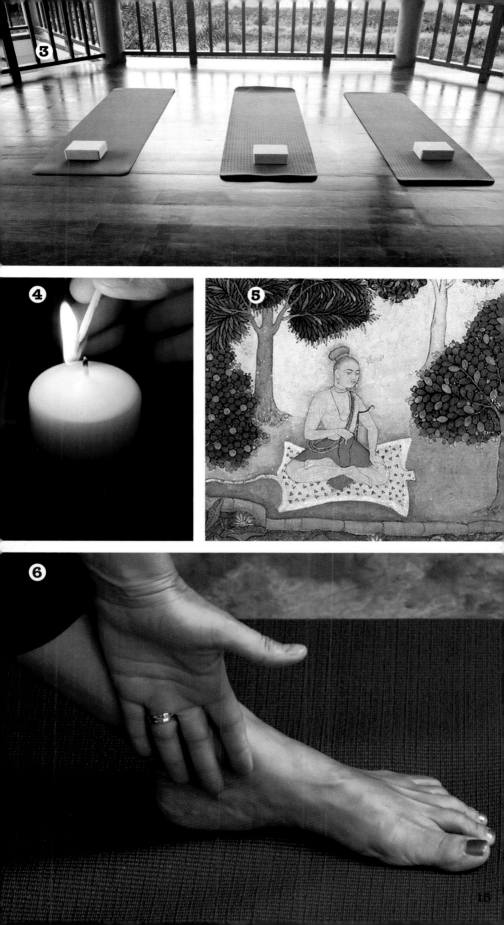

A HISTORY OF YOGA

Yoga and its teachings date back at least to 3000 BC. The practice promoted both physical and spiritual outcomes—the Sanskrit word *yug* means "to yoke together or unite"—and early writings were collected in Hindu scriptures. Today, this versatile discipline is practiced worldwide by lithe athletes, weekend warriors, and golden-agers alike.

Yoga was originally a Hindu spiritual and ascetic discipline that incorporated breath control, meditation, and a series of body postures. Today it is practiced to improve health, achieve a more relaxed state, and elevate consciousness or spirituality. Physically, it is especially useful for increasing flexibility; aligning the skin, muscles, and bones; and strengthening and toning the body.

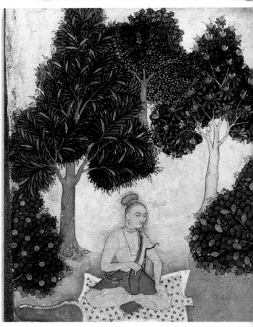

Painting of Yogi seated in a garden

PRE-CLASSICAL YOGA

The first culture to develop yoga was the Indus-Sarasvati civilization of Northern India around 5,000 years ago, though some researchers believe the discipline may date back as far as 10,000 years. The term was first mentioned in the oldest Hindu sacred text, the Rig Veda, a collection of songs, mantras, and rituals. Subsequent developments and refinement in the practice—chronicled by the priest class, the Brahmans, and the mystic seers, the rishis—were collected in the massive compilation of scriptures called the Upanishads. The basic concept behind yoga was the sacrifice of the ego by employing three attributes: self-knowledge;

action, or karma yoga; and wisdom, or jnana yoga. There were, however, many interpretations and manifestations of the practice, which led to an unclear doctrine.

CLASSICAL YOGA

In the second century AD, the clashing, contradictory, or disparate ideas of pre-classical yoga were replaced by a systematic presentation known as Raja yoga, which featured Patanjali's Sutras. Patanjali was a Hindu mystic who organized yoga into "an eight-limbed path" that contained the steps needed to achieve samadhi, or enlightenment. Today Patanjali is considered the father of yoga; many of his sutras still influence modern styles in studios across the globe.

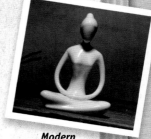

Modern yoga lady

POST-CLASSICAL YOGA

For several centuries after the passing of Patanjali, yoga masters rejected the Vedic teachings and began to concentrate on the physical body as the means to enlightenment and longer life. They created Tantric yoga, with its extreme focus on cleansing the body and mind and slashing the knots that bind us to the physical plane. It was this dual goal, exploring both physical and spiritual connection, that led to the creation of the discipline that once defined yoga in the West—Hatha yoga.

MODERN YOGA

Late in the nineteenth century, Indian yoga masters began a migration to the West in response to sudden interest in the practice. This likely began with the popular lectures on yoga by Swami Vivekananda at the World's Parliament of Religions in Chicago in 1893. His talks included a belief in the universality of all the world's religions. By the 1920s, Hatha yoga had a stronghold in India, but interest in the US was still limited to strict devotees. Then Indra Devi opened her yoga studio in Hollywood, and yoga became an established and accepted form of physical fitness. Western and Indian teachers alike continued to spread the word, opening ashrams and yoga centers, creating new forms of the discipline, and earning millions of new followers.

YOGA FOR EVERYONE

The benefits of yoga are manifold: Many harried career professionals swear by yoga's efficacy as a relaxation technique and laud its ability to "turn down the noise" of busy lives and full schedules. For the athlete, yoga classes offer a chance for recovery after hard workouts at the gym. For seniors, yoga provides low-impact postures that can restore balance, flexibility, and vigor. For couch potatoes who want to get in shape, yoga can be a gradual stepping-stone to more rigorous forms of exercise—or it can be an end in itself.

A SAMPLER OF YOGA STYLES

As the centuries passed, many varieties of yoga evolved, each one placing emphasis on different criteria—continuous movement, precision of body placement, length of time spent in hold, intensity or depth of stretches, or spiritual renewal and psychic restoration.

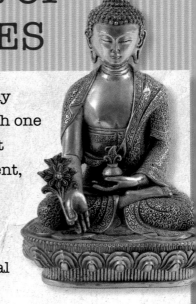

Silver buddha statue

CURRENT CHOICES

Whatever your personal fitness or spiritual goal, you will find that yoga offers something for nearly everyone. The following list covers some of the most popular versions of yoga taught today, along with tips on their target audience and levels of difficulty. You might want to take a few sample classes covering several types of yoga until one clicks. You may also find more than one discipline that works, especially if you desire different results at different times. Always remember that in any level of yoga, the instructor is there to answer questions and guide you safely.

• *Hatha Yoga*. This slower type of yoga, which unifies body and mind, requires the practitioner to hold basic poses for the count of a few breaths. Technically, the Sanskrit term *hatha*—from *ha,* "sun," and *tha*, "moon"—refers to any yoga that teaches physical postures. As a gentle introduction to yoga, it is ideal for beginners.

• *Vinyasa Yoga*. Here the student learns to link continuous movements and breathing in a dance-like, dynamic flow. Transitions are quick and sessions become aerobic; they are often taught to rhythmic music. Vinyasa is especially great for runners and endurance fans.

• *Iyengar Yoga*. This discipline focuses on precise movements and correct body alignment while the poses are held; it utilizes props such as bands, blankets, and blocks. Detail-oriented students will enjoy these classes, but will need at least one beginner session to learn technique. Iyengar works well for older students or those recovering from injuries.

- **Ashtanga Yoga.** This discipline features six sequenced poses that create internal heat as you work your way through them. Some classes have a leader calling out poses; Mysore style requires students to work on their own. Ashtanga is a good fit for anyone who likes movement, routine, and strict guidelines.

- **Bikrim Yoga.** You're guaranteed to sweat as you progress through 26 poses and two breathing exercises in a room heated to 105°F. All classes feature the same 90-minute sequence. Newbies should take things slow at first. Bikrim is best for students who like an established routine and want a really strenuous workout.

- **Hot Yoga.** Like Bikrim, it is performed in a heated studio, but the instructor does not limit the poses to 26. Heated muscles can move into deeper poses, but there is also a risk of overstretching. These classes appeal to those who require the guarantee of a tough, drenching workout.

- **Kundalini Yoga.** With its cultlike following, including many celebrities, this discipline combines challenging mental and physical requirements with controlled breathwork and the inclusion of chanting, singing, and meditating. It appeals greatly to those seeking a spiritual or internal connection to their workout.

- **Yin yoga.** This slow, studied form of yoga incorporates minutes-long holds that target connective tissues and fascia and restore elasticity and length to limbs. It also incorporates meditative qualities that have restorative potential. It is recommended for tense or stressed individuals who need to unwind and stretch.

- **Restorative yoga.** This slow-moving discipline with its longer holds is meant to tap into the parasympathetic nervous system, allowing students to achieve deep relaxation. Props may include bolsters, blankets, and blocks. It works well to reduce insomnia, anxiety, and the jitters, and benefits athletes taking a recovery day.

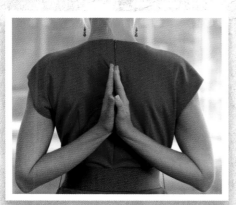

Namaste gesture

 WHAT'S THAT MEAN?
KUNDALINI

In yoga, "kundalini" is latent female or primal energy, often represented as a serpent coiled around the base of the spinal column. When this energy is stimulated, it uncoils, and you may experience a transformative "kundalini awakening."

COMMON YOGA TERMS

Many of the terms used in yoga are based on Sanskrit, the classical language of India, especially of ancient Hindu scriptures and epic poems. When yoga terms are pronounced properly, distinct inhalations and exhalations result, similar to those used in meditative mantras.

Ashram: a hermitage; a monastic community or a religious retreat, especially in India and Southeast Asia.

Asana: a physical posture of yoga.

Ashtanga: the eight-limbed yogic path.

Ayurveda: ancient Indian science of health.

Bakasana: Sanskrit term for the basic Crane pose or Crow pose, where the folded torso is balanced above the arms and the bent knees rest upon bent elbows. Also called *Kakasana*.

Bakti: devotion, as in Bakti yoga.

Bandha: an internal lock used for controlling the energy inside the body during yoga; the three locks taught in Hatha yoga are the root lock, the abdominal lock, and the throat lock.

Buddha: the enlightened one; in Buddhism, refers to Siddhartha Gautama, a spiritual teacher during the sixth to fourth centuries BC who became enlightened.

Chakra: an energy center; the human body has seven—root, sacrum, solar plexus, heart, throat, third eye, and crown—and each one is associated with a color, element, syllable, significance, and so forth.

Dharma: truth; the path of truth; the teachings of the Buddha.

Dosha: a physical body type; in ayurvedic medicine there are three: *pitta* (fire), *vata* (wind), and *kapha* (earth).

Drishti: a gazing point used during asanas.

Guru: spiritual teacher or master; literally "one who illuminates the darkness."

WHAT'S THAT MEAN? NIYAMA AND YAMA

These comprise two sets of five living principles that make up the ethical and moral foundation of yoga. Niyamas include Sauca (purity), Santosha (contentment), Tapas (burning enthusiasm), Svadhyaya (self-study) and Ishvarapranidhana (celebration of the spiritual). Yamas include Satya (truth), Ahimsa (nonviolence), Asteya (not stealing), Bramacharya (self-control and sexual responsibility), and Aparigraha (not grasping).

Kirtan: a community gathering that includes chanting, music, and meditation.

Mantra: a repeated sound that facilitates meditation; a sacred thought or prayer. Can be sounds, syllables, words, or groups of words that create a positive transformation.

Meditation: focusing the mind through breathing in order to reach a deeper level of consciousness.

Mudra: a hand gesture that influences one's energies. Palms are pressed together in prayer position for anjali mudra, and forefinger and thumb are touching in gyana mudra.

Namaste: "I bow to you," a greeting used among friends, or among yoga instructors and students. More subtly it says: "I honor the universe that resides inside you. When I am in my inner universe and you are in yours, there is only one of us."

Neutral Position: In the spine, this means all three natural curves—cervical (neck), thoracic (middle), and lumbar (lower)—are present and in proper alignment. If the skin of your neck creases during a pose, it is out of natural alignment.

Om or Aum: considered the first sound of creation, it is frequently chanted during meditation or before, during, or after yoga classes.

Prana: life energy; chi; qi.

Pranyama: breath awareness; control of breathing to improve inner stillness.

Samadhi: a state of complete enlightenment.

Savasana: the Sanskrit term for Corpse pose; typically, the final relaxation pose at the end of a yoga class.

Shakti: female energy.

Shanti: peace; the term is often chanted three times.

Shiva: male energy; a Hindu deity.

Surya Namskar: sun salutations; a system of yoga poses performed in a series or flow.

Sutras: classical Indian texts.

Swami: defined as a "master," a Hindu ascetic or religious leader, especially a senior member of a religious order.

Tantra: the yoga of union between mind and body.

Ujjayi breathing: also called Hissing Breath or Victorious Breath, involves fully expanding the lungs and puffing out the chest during yoga poses, especially during Vinyasa-style classes.

Yoga: from the Sanskrit yug or "to unite"; an ancient practice that incorporates breathing practices, physical postures, meditation, and philosophy in order to achieve enlightenment.

Yogi/yogini: a male/female practitioner of yoga.

A DEDICATED SPACE

While it is always worthwhile to attend yoga classes—you'll improve your technique, make new friends, and feel a sense of accomplishment—it doesn't take a lot to carve out a home sanctuary where you can practice yoga . . . or simply sit and relax.

Among the benefits of creating a home yoga studio are being able to indulge yourself in the practice whenever the mood strikes (or the stress strikes!); providing yourself and your family a dedicated space without household clutter, stray toys, or jarring noises; and giving yourself the gift of privacy, if you so choose, away from the hectic pace of family life. Once you have a yoga area, it probably won't be long before you are using that space for other spiritual pursuits, such as meditation, chanting, chime therapy, or other restorative practices. Plus, many people who have created and begun to regularly use a yoga "den" report that it has become a catalyst for other positive changes in their lives—seeking new job opportunities, enrolling in additional classes or schooling, or focusing on building better personal relationships or more meaningful friendships.

WHAT YOU WILL NEED
Look around your home for a space you can convert. If you are a homeowner, investigate the basement, finished attic, or a heated garage. An old kid's playroom or outgrown nursery could be perfect. A few lucky people may have the right climate to create an outdoor space, perhaps under a carport or partially covered patio, and take advantage of fresh air and natural

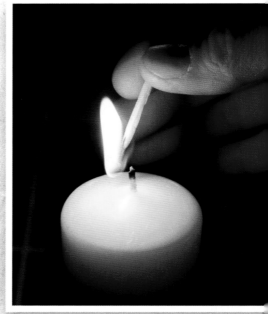

light. Apartment dwellers may have to take over a corner of the bedroom or part of the living room to create their space, but it will be worth it in the end. If you accessorize it nicely—and roll up your mat when you are done—it will become a welcoming spot, whatever its purpose.

Ideally, your yoga studio should have enough floor space to place two mats three feet apart, and enough room to house a small but comfy chair and a small desk or table. A CD or MP3 player on the table can provide soft music, and a DVD player and monitor can be used for watching instructional videos. The lighting should be soft, but not too dark. Overhead lighting tends to be harsh, so opt for floor or table lamps. If you have the freedom to paint the area, soft pastels (like sea greens or pale slate blues) are very relaxing—deep reds, oranges, and yellows are not. Hanging a wall mirror also makes sense, especially if you want to practice new poses.

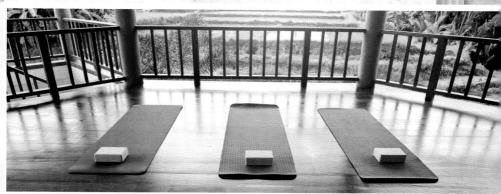

DAILY ACTIVITIES

You'll be surprised how many reasons you'll find to visit your quiet space in the course of a day in addition to the time spent there practicing your regular yoga routines.

• First thing in the morning, energize your body with seven sun salutations.
• Practice your breathing and facial exercises.
• Pop in a DVD about another discipline, perhaps tai chi or Pilates.
• Indulge in craft making, create a vision board, or join the kids on the floor for some finger painting.
• If you're feeling sore, ease the pain with gentle poses that target those tender areas.
• Instead of lounging on the couch on the weekends, invite your significant other or best friend to join you for some basic poses or light stretching.
• Use the solitude to meditate or to work out the solution to a problem or conflict.
• Bring a good book and a glass of wine or cup of tea to your cozy chair.
• When you get home from a busy day, set a timer and relax on your mat for 15 minutes.
• Do some light stretching before bedtime to ease away the kinks and relax.

ACCESSORIES FOR SERENITY

Once you have outfitted your yoga space with a few small pieces of furniture and some soft lighting, you will need to bring in the proper equipment or props and some personalized accessories that will help create an air of tranquility.

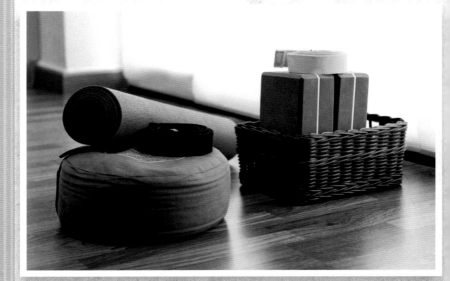

PERSONAL TOUCHES

In addition to bringing sounds, scents, and artwork into your sanctuary, let your imagination roam outdoors and take advantage of natural objects to embellish your yoga space.

• Use the resonant tones of bells, Tibetan singing bowls, chimes, and gongs to help you relax before or after your session.
• Keep a selection of DVDs that offer different levels of yoga instruction.
• Start a collection of CDs that feature Indian, ethnic, or inspirational music.
• Hang up your favorite artwork, meaningful images, tapestries, wind chimes, or soothing spiritual objects such as dream catchers, Russian icons, or Mexican *retablos*. Remember that Swami Vivekananda taught the universality of all religions.

- Place natural objects such as shells, sea glass, crystals and minerals, feathers, nests, and colored glass bottles around your space.
- Use flameless votive or pillar candles for safety, and place them in ceramic, glass, or brass holders or Asian-style lanterns.
- If there is a window in your space, try adding oxygen-expelling plants

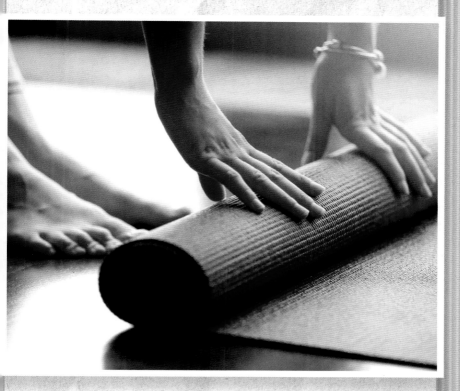

to cleanse the air and brighten the view. If there is no window nearby, try plants with low-light requirements, such as spider plants and asparagus ferns.

- If your space abuts a busy part of your home, invest in an inexpensive screen and unfold it when you are practicing or trying to relax. You can also ask younger family members to respect a 15-minute quiet time—before chaos reigns again.

BENEFICIAL PROPERTIES

Essential oil diffusers can create an aromatic ambience as well as enhance your mental state. A number of beneficial oils are able to stimulate the mind-body connection, especially when combined with thumb and forefinger mudras. Consider the virtues of stress-relieving bergamot; depression-easing patchouli; reviving and grounding sandalwood; uplifting lemon; protective and healing frankincense; or anger-reducing Roman chamomile. You can also burn incense cones or joss sticks in the same mood-elevating scents.

ASANAS FOR RELAXATION

Although most yoga poses are not normally aerobic, some intermediate or advanced ones can be taxing to perform. So it's nice to know that there are a number of gentler poses that offer relaxation, relief from tension and pain, and even renewed energy.

CHILD'S POSE

This stress-relieving beginner pose, also known as Balasana, stretches the spine, hips, buttocks, thighs, and ankles. It gently relaxes the front muscles of the body while passively stretching the posterior muscles of the torso. It also fights fatigue and eases neck pain.

• Kneel on the floor with your hips over your knees. Bring your feet together and fold the torso onto your legs, while elongating your neck and spine.
• Stretch your arms forward, palms facing down.
• Widen your shoulders as you place your forehead on the floor. Hold pose from one to five minutes depending on your comfort level.
Tip: Inhaling to the back of your rib cage allows your back to form a dome; keep your neck extended with your crown facing forward.

EXTENDED PUPPY POSE

Also known as Uttana Shishosana, this beginnger's pose is a combination of Child's Pose and Downward Facing Dog (page 28). It stretches the shoulders, arms, hips, and upper back, and increases flexibility in the spine. It calms the mind, energizes the body, and can also relieve tension and insomnia.

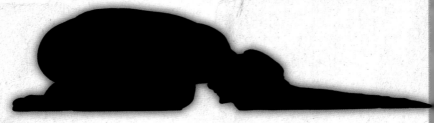

- Kneel with your knees directly below your hips. With arms shoulder-width apart, bend forward onto your hands and knees.
- As you exhale, lower chest toward floor, press hips back, and slide arms forward, keeping palms flat.
- Ease your forehead onto the floor while stretching arms forward and spine in both directions. Hold for 30 seconds to 1 minute.

Tip: Slightly arch upper back to stretch shoulders and spine; don't rest elbows on floor or let middle of torso droop.

EASY POSE

This beginner pose, known as Sukhasana, is used to strengthen the back, broaden the chest and collarbone, and stretch the knees and ankles; it also opens the hips, groin, and outer thigh muscles. Sitting upright in this pose with your spine aligned has the added benefit of calming the brain and reducing stress and anxiety.

- Sit up straight on your mat and extend your legs in front of your body, as in Staff Pose (page 28).
- Cross your legs in front of you at the shins and widen your knees as you place each foot beneath the opposite knee.
- Fold both legs in toward your torso and rest your forearms along each thigh. Hold the posture for as long as possible and then switch leg positions.

Tip: You can position your fingers in gyana mudra, touching forefingers and thumb, or place hands in prayer mudra, pressing palm to palm at chest height.

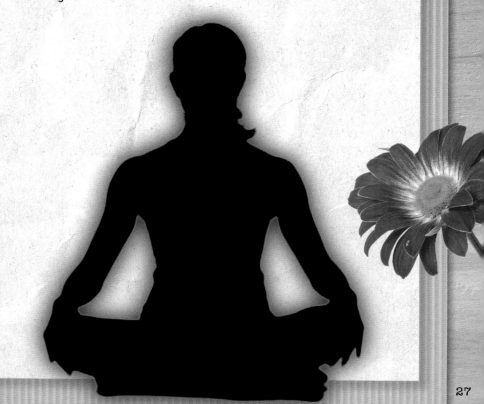

ASANAS FOR RELAXATION

STAFF POSE

This beginner pose, called Dandasana, offers a range of benefits: It helps to improve posture, strengthen back muscles, and lengthen the spine. It can relieve complications of the reproductive system, expand the shoulders and chest, increase resistance to back and hip problems, and even help to calm an overburdened brain.

• Sit on the floor with your back straight and legs extended from hip, arms resting at your sides.

• Press down with your sit bones and extend the crown of your head toward the ceiling.

• Flex your feet and press outward with your heels. Hold as long as you can, or for at least 5 to 10 breaths.

Tip: Inhale deeply while stretching your legs, and exhale deeply while broadening the shoulders and opening the chest. Exhale again after releasing the pose.

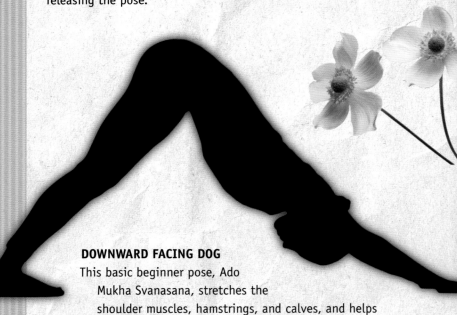

DOWNWARD FACING DOG

This basic beginner pose, Ado Mukha Svanasana, stretches the shoulder muscles, hamstrings, and calves, and helps to strengthen the hands, wrists, arms, and legs. It can decrease back pain by strengthening the spine and shoulder girdle; it also calms the mind and relieves mild depression.

• Kneel on hands and knees with knees positioned below your hips and your toes bent forward.
• As you press your heels and palms to the floor, straighten your knees and elbows and angle your body so that your buttocks are elevated above your torso.
• Keep your head lowered between your arms and do not round your spine. Hold for 30 seconds to 2 minutes.
Tip: It helps to first practice this pose with knees bent and heels up. Avoid this pose if you suffer from carpal tunnel syndrome.

LEGS UP THE WALL POSE

The beginner pose known as Viparita Karani is one of the most nourishing, grounding, and calming postures found in yoga, and one that many students turn to when they feel tired, overwhelmed, or stressed. It reduces edema in the lower limbs, eases weary leg muscles, and offers the benefits of inversion without all the effort.

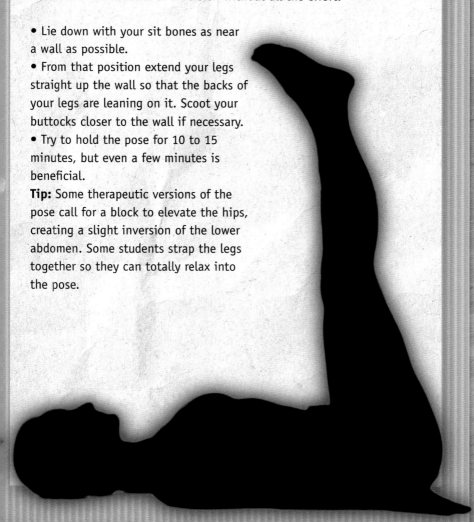

• Lie down with your sit bones as near a wall as possible.
• From that position extend your legs straight up the wall so that the backs of your legs are leaning on it. Scoot your buttocks closer to the wall if necessary.
• Try to hold the pose for 10 to 15 minutes, but even a few minutes is beneficial.
Tip: Some therapeutic versions of the pose call for a block to elevate the hips, creating a slight inversion of the lower abdomen. Some students strap the legs together so they can totally relax into the pose.

ASANAS FOR STRETCHING

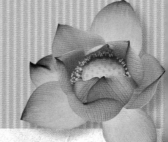

The medical link between wellness and flexibility has been well established. The more freely you can move, the easier it is to stay fit as you age. Yoga stretches specifically target the large muscle groups that allow you to achieve and maintain flexibility.

SEATED FORWARD BEND

This beginner pose, known as Paschimattanasana, is good for stretching the shoulders, spine, and hamstrings. It is known to stimulate digestion and reduce stress or anxiety, and can help to lower blood pressure. Do not attempt this pose if you have back problems or diarrhea.

• From Staff Pose (page 28), rock back and forth slightly to move your sit bones back.
• Inhale and raise your arms straight up from shoulders. Exhale and stretch your chest forward, bending from the hips.
• Bring your abdomen to your thighs, your forehead to your shins, and reach down to grasp your soles or your ankles. Try not to round your back or force the torso down. To help you bend at first, place a folded blanket under your buttocks.
• Hold for 1 to 3 minutes.
Tip: Make sure to elongate your spine from neck to hips. Keep the neck in neutral position.

INTENSE SIDE STRETCH

This intermediate pose, also known as Parsvottanasana, stretches the shoulders, spine, and hamstrings as it strengthens the leg muscles. It also gives a boost to digestion. Avoid if you have high blood pressure or suffer from spine or back issues.

• Begin in Mountain Pose (page 44); bring your hands behind your back and position them in reverse prayer hands.
• As you exhale, step your left foot forward three feet and turn the rear foot out slightly as you turn your torso slightly to the right.
• Tuck tailbone in and lower torso from waist toward left thigh. Hold 15 to 30 seconds then switch legs.
Tip: Keep back flat, chest tucked in to thigh, and neck in neutral position; make sure both feet remain flat on floor.

BRIDGE POSE

This versatile beginner pose, also called the Setu Bandha Sarvangasana, has a number of variations. It opens the shoulders and chest, strengthens the thighs and buttocks, and stretches the neck, thorax, and back. It is known to aid digestion and relieve stress.

• Lie supine with your arms at your sides and your knees bent; slide your heels toward your body.
• Press the soles of your feet down and raise your buttocks. With thighs and feet parallel, inhale and press down with your arms as you lift your hips and raise your torso from the floor. Use buttocks and legs to elevate torso.
• Hold for 30 to 60 seconds.
Tip: Roll your shoulders under as your torso rises; keep knees directly over heels. Don't tuck your chin into your chest.

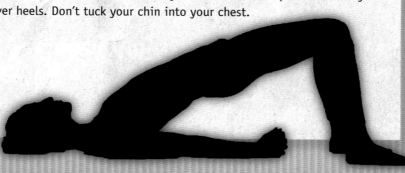

ASANAS FOR STRETCHING

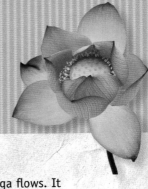

TRIANGLE POSE

This pose is a familiar part of most standing yoga flows. It lengthens the muscles at the side of the waist and extends both the hamstrings and hips. It also improves stability and decreases stress. Do not perform if you have low blood pressure or suffer from recurring headaches.

• Stand with your arms straight out from your shoulders. Step your right foot back several feet and turn it slightly outward.
• Bend your torso forward from the waist over your extended leg until it is parallel with the floor.
• Lower your right hand to rest on your right shin as you turn your head to face the ceiling. (Those with neck problems should gaze forward or at the ground.)
• Hold for 30 seconds before standing upright and switching sides.
Tip: Keep arms and legs straight throughout this pose. Inhale as you lengthen your spine, then exhale as you twist forward from the waist.

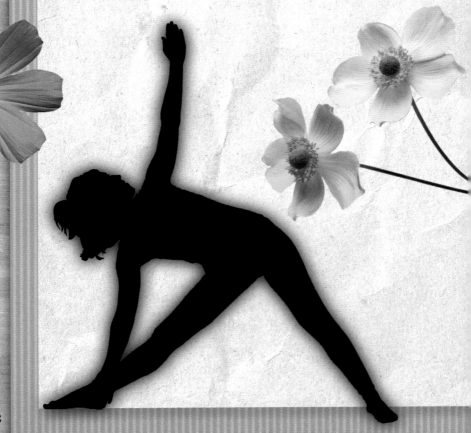

RECLINING BIG TOE POSE

Also called Supta Padangusthasana, this easy pose is popular in studios around the world. It helps to strengthen the knees while it stretches the hips, thighs, hamstrings, and groin. It is believed to benefit the prostate gland, improve digestion, and ease backache, sciatica, and menstrual pain. It is not advisable if you've recently had hip surgery.

• Lie supine and raise your right leg over your torso, rotating your leg so that your knee faces your armpit.
• Grab your elevated big toe with the fingers of your right hand while left hand clasps top of left thigh. Straighten your leg enough to feel the stretch, mainly in your hamstring.
• Hold for 15 to 30 seconds, then repeat with opposite leg.

Tip: Use a strap around your foot if you can't reach your big toe. Keep buttocks firmly on the mat and keep neck elongated.

HALF FROG POSE

The Ardha Bhekasana is known to open up the chest, shoulders, and thighs, work the hip muscles and thigh flexors, and improve the flexibility of the back. It not only prepares the student for back-bend poses, it's also a beneficial stretch for runners and cyclists.

• Lie prone with palms flat on floor, and press down to raise your torso.
• As you soften the top of the right thigh and shift your right side slightly to the front, bend your right leg.
• Cross your left hand in front of your body, then reach back to your right foot with your right hand, fingers facing forward, and use your palm to press your foot gently toward the outside of your right hip.
• Hold for seconds to 2 minutes, before switching sides.

Tip: Keep bent knee aligned with hip. If there is knee pain instead of tension in thigh, ease up on pose. Don't slump down into shoulder or forward arm.

ASANAS FOR STRETCHING

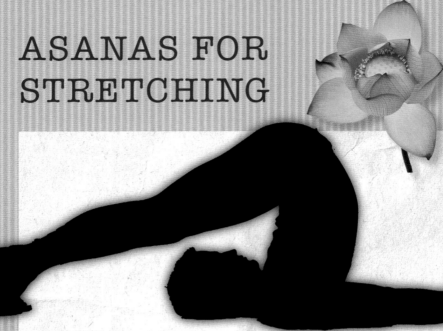

PLOW POSE

This intermediate pose, also known as Halasana, works well for soothing headaches or backaches, relieving stress, and aiding digestion. It especially targets the muscles of the chest, shoulder, and scapula.

• Lie flat with your arms at your sides, knees bent. Raise your legs off the floor by pressing down with your arms for leverage. Then elevate your back, using your bent arms to support your spine.
• Bring your legs over your head and touch your toes to the floor behind your crown. Straighten arms along floor for stability.
• While keeping your torso perpendicular to the floor, hold the pose for 1 to 5 minutes.
Tip: Place a folded blanket under your shoulders to ease your spine. Don't flop your legs down into the pose—lower them in a controlled manner.

KNEES TO CHEST POSE

This beginner pose, also called Apanasana, is a great way to stretch and stabilize the lower back and hips—it can even ease low-back pain, sciatica, spinal stenosis, and disc herniation. It is also beneficial as an aid to digestion, and as a means to reduce anger, tension, and high blood pressure. Avoid this pose if you are pregnant or have recently had knee surgery.
• Lie supine on the floor; exhale and draw your knees toward your chest

until your thighs are nearly parallel with the floor.

• Place your hands over the front of your knees as you extend your neck away from your shoulders. Flatten back and shoulders on floor as you gently draw knees closer.

• Hold for 30 seconds to one minute.

Tip: While in pose, don't tense your back or leg muscles. Flexible advanced students can wrap their arms around their knees and grasp opposite elbows with each hand.

GARLAND POSE

This deep squat, also called Malasana, opens the hips—which stimulates your metabolism—stretches the groin and lower back, and strengthens the ankles and tightens the belly. This pose makes an excellent prep for the more complex balancing Crow Pose (page 38). It is not advised for those with knee problems.

• Begin in Mountain Pose (page 44) with feet slightly wider than hip distance apart; turn toes out like a ballerina.

• Bend knees deeply, easing down into squat position with your hips lower than your knees. Keep knees pointing in same direction as toes to protect vulnerable joints.

• Lean your chest forward, fold palms together at chest height, and press your elbows against your inner thighs to separate them and lengthen the spine.

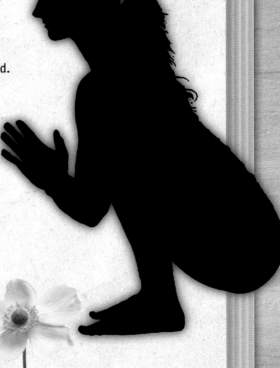

• Hold for a count of 5 breaths, straighten legs as you inhale, and come up into a passive forward fold.

Tip: If you can't comfortably keep your heels on the ground, place a folded blanket beneath them.

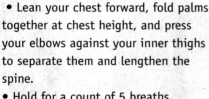

ASANAS FOR STRETCHING

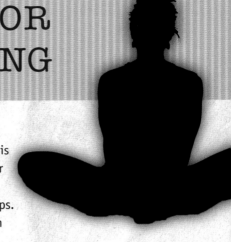

BOUND ANGLE POSE

Also known as the Tailor Pose, this beginner pose stretches the inner thighs, groin, and knees. It can also help to ease menstrual cramps. Do not attempt if you suffer from groin pain or knee problems.

• Sit on the floor with your legs extended, then bend your knees and bring your legs up close to your chest.
• While exhaling, lower your thighs outward toward the floor; use your hands to keep the outsides of both feet on the floor.
• Sit up straight, creating a straight line from sit bones to shoulders. Keep your spine neutral by drawing your lower torso up and spreading your weight over your sit bones.
• Hold pose for 1 to 4 minutes.
Tip: If there is initial pain while in position, sit on a folded blanket or lean forward from the chest. Don't push your knees down with your hands.

FIRELOG POSE

Also called Agnistambhasana, this intermediate pose strengthens the legs and calves, opens the hips, stretches the groin and buttock muscles, and stimulates the abdominal organs. The pose eases anxiety, tension, and stress by calming the mind. Avoid this pose if you suffer from groin or knee issues.

• Starting from Easy Pose (page 27), place the right ankle on the left knee so that the right foot is on outside of left knee.
• Tuck left ankle under right knee so that both shins are stacked. Flex your toes. (If it causes you discomfort to tuck the bottom ankle under the top knee, tuck it back toward the hip.)
• Elevate your torso on your sit bones, exhale, and allow your hips to open.
• Hold pose for 1 to 3 minutes, then repeat with leg positions reversed.
Tip: Make sure your legs are

rotating out from your hips, not your knees. Do not allow your feet or ankles to pronate or collapse inward.

STANDING WARRIOR 1

This is one of three Standing Warrior Poses; it is useful for creating strength and stability in the ankles, back, and thighs, as well as thoroughly stretching the front of the body. The posture allows for a deep expansion of the chest and lungs. This pose energizes the body and restores calm and focus.

• Stand upright with arms at sides; lunge by stepping your left foot three feet forward in front of right foot. Keep toes of right foot angled outward.
• As you exhale, bend left knee and lower hips, keeping your shoulders directly above your hips.
• Raise your arms straight up from your shoulders so that torso and arms form a line perpendicular to the floor.
• Hold the pose for 2 to 5 breaths, then step right foot forward.
Tip: Keep the soles of both feet firmly grounded; from your fingertips, pull along your arms and spine. Do not twist the knee of your back leg.

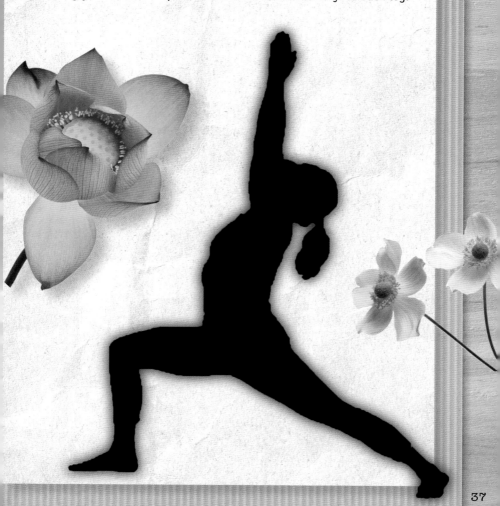

ASANAS FOR STRENGTH AND BALANCE

CROW POSE

This intermediate posture, also called Crane Pose or Bakasana, not only strengthens the shoulders, arms, abdominals, and wrists, but also improves balance and stability. It can be used as a learning tool for balancing on your arms during other, more complex, poses.

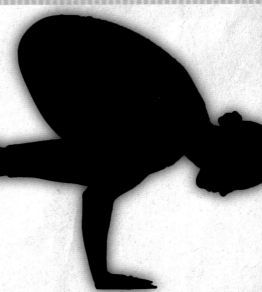

• From squatting in Garland Pose (page 35), lean your torso forward while placing your hands flat in front of you, fingers spread.
• Bend you elbows and place your bent knees against your upper arms. Shift body up onto tiptoes, and slide your shins along your upper arms.
• Shift your weight onto your wrists and raise one foot at a time from the ground. Totter until you find the right balance. Hold for 20 seconds to 1 minute.
Tip: Gazing at one spot on the floor can help maintain balance. Try not to "leap" into the pose, but assume it gradually. Do not drop your head down.

FISH POSE

Also known as Matasyasana, this pose supposedly allows one to float like a fish if practiced in the water. It can help improve posture and strengthen the upper back and the neck. It also stretches the throat, navel, abdominals, and the intercostal muscles found between the ribs.

- As you lie supine, slip your flattened hands, palms down, beneath your buttocks.
- Bend your elbows as you press down with your forearms and raise your chest in order to arch your back. Be careful not to lift your hips.
- Keeping your weight on your elbows, ease your head back so that the top rests on the floor.
- Hold pose for 15 to 30 seconds.

Tip: Keep forearms close to the body; legs can be straight or bent. Avoid putting weight on the head or neck.

LOCUST POSE

Also known as Salabhansana, this beginner pose stretches the hip flexors, the chest, and the abdominals, and can strengthen the spine, buttocks, arms, and legs. Like other back-bend poses, it helps to stimulate digestion. Many students use it to prep for more demanding back-bend poses.

- Lie prone on the floor, arms at your sides, palms facing down.
- Turn your legs inward slightly, so that your toes point at the floor.
- As you inhale, squeeze your buttocks and lift your head, arms, and legs, as though your are imitating Superman.
- Use your pelvis and abdominal muscles to stabilize you as you raise your limbs as high as possible, while keeping neck in neutral position.
- Hold for 30 to 60 seconds; repeat several times.

Tip: Make sure to open your chest and elongate your neck to extend the stretch along your entire spine. Try not to bend your knees.

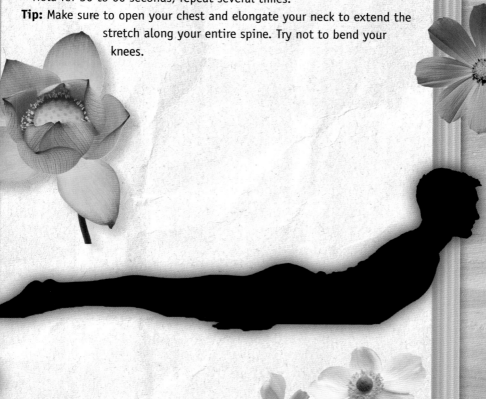

ASANAS FOR STRENGTH AND BALANCE

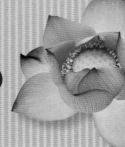

FOUR LIMB STAFF POSE

Also called the Chaturanga or the Low Plank, this posture strengthens the abdominals, the triceps, the pectorals, the shoulder blades, and the wrists. If you have trouble staying parallel to the ground, keep your knees on the floor at first.

• From plank pose, open up your chest, widen your shoulders, and tuck in your sit bones.
• While exhaling, turn your legs in a bit, and lower your torso until your upper arms are parallel to your spine. Try to position your body in a straight line.
• Keep elbows tucked in and abdomen tight; hold the pose for 15 to 30 seconds.

Tip: You can maintain better stability if you tighten your buttocks and hold in your abdomen. Keep your neck in neutral position, and don't hunch your shoulders.

WARRIOR 2

One of three Standing Warrior Poses, this one often occurs in sequences before Warrior 1 (page 37). It is important for establishing inner strength and stamina while honing stability in the legs, ankles, hips, back, and shoulders. It opens both the chest and hips, stimulates circulation, and sends energy throughout the body.

• Step your left foot back about 3 feet and turn your left foot out at a 90-degree angle.

- Slowly bend your right knee as you begin to lower your hips.
- Raise your torso so that your spine is extended while your shoulders remain directly above your hips.
- Raise your arms straight out so they are parallel to the floor.
- Hold the pose for at least 5 breaths before repeating with the opposite leg extended.

Tip: Keep both feet firmly on the ground and try not to lean forward over your hips or arch your lower back.

UPWARD FACING DOG

Part of the Sun Salutation series of poses, Urdu Mukha Svansana lifts and opens the chest, and lengthens and strengthens the anterior muscles of the back, buttocks, thighs, arms, and legs.

- Lie prone on floor with palms flat and forearms perpendicular to floor.
- Press palms into floor and extend arms as you roll your sholders up and back. Extend chest forward, arch your back, and raise the crown of your head toward the ceiling.
- As you inhale, slightly raise legs and thighs from the floor by pressing down with the tops of your feet. Hold pose for 15 to 30 seconds, then exhale as you lower yourself to the floor.

Tip: Make sure that shoulders, elbows, and wrists align as you push upward. Keep buttocks firm but not clenched. Be careful not to round shoulders, push out ribs, or let thighs droop.

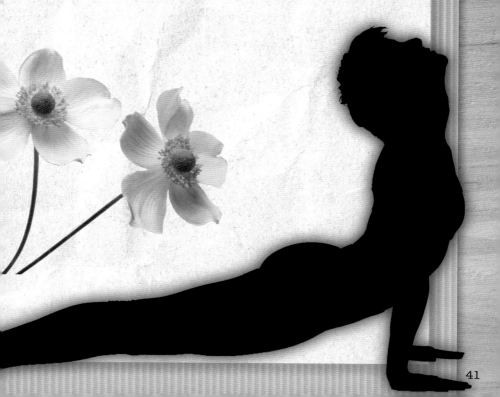

ASANAS FOR STRENGTH AND BALANCE

WIDE ANGLE SEATED BEND

This intermediate pose is also called Upavistha Konasana. It stretches the groin muscles, the glutes, and the hamstrings and also strengthens the back. Make sure to keep your buttocks firmly on the floor; do not let them roll forward. As you increase the flexibility in your waist and lower back, you will be able to lean forward without shifting off the floor.

• From Staff Pose (page 28), spread legs wide apart, turning your thighs slightly outward. Flex your feet.
• Place hands behind buttocks and push them forward to widen leg position. Press your sit bones and the back of your thighs to the floor.
• With hands in front of you, exhale and bend forward from the hips, and walk your hands out and away from you. Keeping back flat, lower torso to the floor. Keep your eyes forward.
• Stretch hands and torso forward without rounding back. Hold for 30 seconds to 2 minutes.
Tip: Keep toes pointed up to the ceiling during this pose; don't lean forward from the waist, but instead bend from the hips.

TWISTING CHAIR POSE

This standing pose, known as Parivrtta Utkanasana, stretches the spine, shoulders, and chest, while strengthening the mid and lower back, thighs, buttocks, and hips. It also stretches the side muscles and tones internal organs such as the GI tract and kidneys. This can help to detoxify the body, improving overall health.

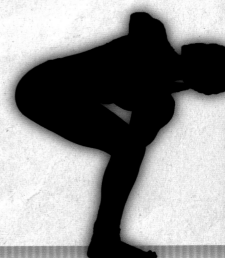

- Stand with feet together and bend your knees until your hips are level with them.
- Raise your arms up and twist your torso to the right, raising one shoulder. Press your left elbow on the outside of the right knee.
- Press palms together in prayer mudra and bring your gaze upward.
- Hold for 10 to 20 seconds before switching sides.

Tip: To maintain balance, keep your weight on your heels rather than on the balls of your feet. Don't arch or stiffen your back, but instead keep a slight curve in the lower back.

BOW POSE

This intermediate pose, also called Dhanuranasana, stretches the abdominals, hip flexors, and quads as it strengthens the spine and stimulates the GI tract. By changing the direction of your grip—palms on inner or outer ankle bones—you can also work a different set of muscles. The pose should be avoided by anyone with back problems, high or low blood pressure, or a headache.

- Lie prone on the floor with arms relaxed at sides. Place chin on the floor.
- Exhale and bend your knees, bringing your feet to your buttocks; reach back and grasp the outside of your ankles.
- Inhale to lift your chest from the floor, raise your ankles up with feet flexed, and shift your weight to your abdominals as your body arches. Keep head in neutral position.
- Hold for 15 to 30 seconds as you take short, controlled breaths.

Tip: Make sure to keep your elevated knees the same width as your hips. Don't rock your weight back onto your pelvis.

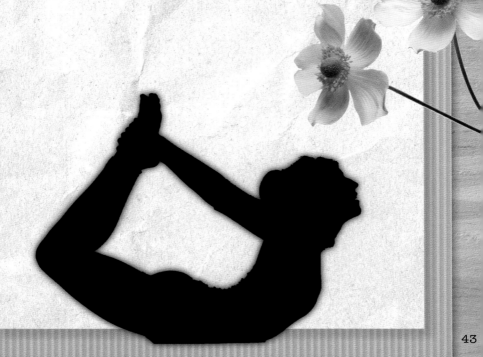

ASANAS FOR STRENGTH AND BALANCE

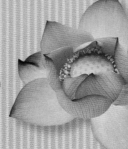

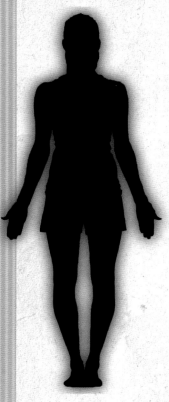

MOUNTAIN POSE

This is the foundational pose from which all standing and inverted poses flow. It targets the core and the muscles of the thighs.

• Stand with feet together, arms at sides. Press weight evenly over balls of feet and arches.
• Bring pelvis into neutral position, with hip bones pointing neither down nor up.
• Elongate your torso and shift shoulder blades toward back of waist.
• As you lengthen your spine, hold the pose for one minute.

Tip: Align your ears, shoulders, hips, and heels. Stop pose if you become dizzy.

TREE POSE

This pose helps to build strength and balance along the thigh muscles and core; it stretches the thighs, groin, torso, and shoulders.

• Stand straight, with feet together. Shift weight onto right foot.
• Use your right hand to reach down and grasp your right ankle.
• Raise your right foot until it is resting against your upper left thigh.
• Center yourself and place your hands in prayer position in front of your chest.
• Try to maintain balance for at least 10 seconds. Repeat using left foot.
Tip: Foot can rest above or below the supporting knee. Do not turn out the supporting foot or the knee will misalign.

HALF MOON POSE

This standing pose will tax your abdominals and leg muscles and improve balance. It also opens the chest, groin, and hamstrings.

• Stand straight up, right foot forward, arms extended straight out from your sides.
• Shift your weight onto your right foot, bending forward at the waist and raising your left leg behind you, foot flexed.
• Once your back is parallel to the ground, twist your torso and reach down with left arm so that your palm touches the floor; raise your right arm straight above you.
• Either keep eyes looking forward or turn head to gaze up.
• Hold for 30 seconds to 1 minute, then switch legs.
Tip: Lengthen the raised leg by pulling outward from your head; do not perform if you have low blood pressure, headaches, or diarrhea.

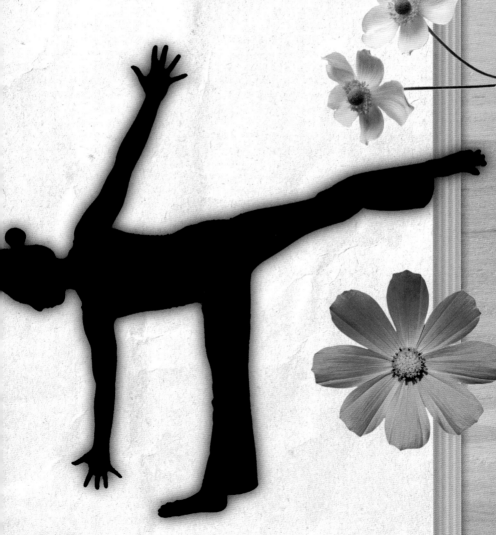

WHOLE BODY POSES

There are a number of beginner or intermediate poses that have the advantage of strengthening or stretching a wide variety of muscles or body parts. Besides the three shown here, you might want to also try Forearm Plank, Boat Pose, and Locust Pose (page 39).

PLANK POSE
Although it looks intimidating, the Plank, or Phalakasana, is a beginner/intermediate pose. It strengthens the wrists, arms, legs, and all the core muscles, including the abdomen, chest, and lower back. Two tips for success are keeping your body weight distributed evenly and extending your legs right down to the heels. The Plank is also a great way to improve your sense of balance in preparation for other, more difficult, poses.

• From Downward Facing Dog (page 28), walk the torso forward so that your wrists are directly under your shoulders, with your legs extended behind you and your toes curled to the front.
• Widen your shoulder position and tighten your legs.
• Hold for 30 seconds to 1 minute.
Tip: Ideally, your body should form a straight line from head to heels; clench buttocks and tighten abdominals to aid stability. Don't allow your hips to sag or your shoulders to hunch.

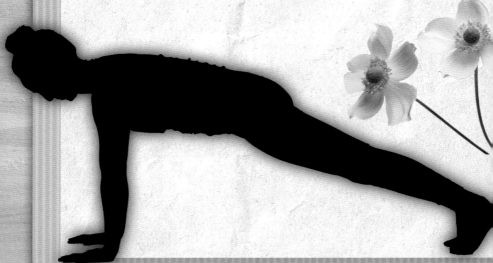

SIDE PLANK

This beginner pose, called Vasisthasana, calls for you to balance on one arm, so it strengthens the wrists, arms, and shoulders, as well as the belly and legs. Do not attempt this pose if you have wrist or elbow problems or issues with your shoulders.

- From Plank Pose, shift your weight to the outside of your right foot and onto your right arm. Raise left shoulder up and back.
- Stack the left foot over the right, bring legs together, and straighten them.
- As you exhale, raise your left arm up toward the ceiling, fingers reaching, while gazing at your fingertips.
- Hold for 15 to 30 seconds, then repeat pose on the opposite side.

Tip: Your ankles, hips, and shoulders should form one straight line, as should the extension from left wrist to right wrist through your shoulders.

EXTENDED HAND TO FOOT POSE

This pose, known as Tadasana, helps to improve both balance and flexibility in much of the body. Make sure to focus on firming up the supporting leg and elongating your spine before raising the leg.

> ### KEEP IT SIMPLE
> The full version of the Side Plank calls for the upper leg to be held perpendicular to the floor. The modified version shown here falls more within the scope of most students.

- Begin in Mountain Pose (page 44) and shift your weight onto your right foot; raise your left knee toward your belly while placing your right hand on your right hip for balance.
- Reach down and grab your big toe with your left hand; wrap two fingers around inside of toe, thumb around the outside.
- Rotate right thigh in slightly, firm up your grounded leg, and, as you exhale, extend your left leg until knee is straight.
- Find the proper balance, then hold for 1 to 5 breaths; switch legs.

Tip: Keep spine long and shoulders in line with hips. Do not let your hip tilt up as your raise your leg; don't let your knee lock or tilt inward.

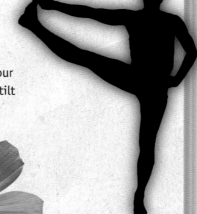

COOL DOWN POSES

Some yoga postures can actually help lower your body temperature, reducing the thermal energy caused by exertion. Use these poses to cool down after a demanding yoga class or try them to chill out on a hot, humid day.

BUTTERFLY POSE

This simple pose, also called Baddha Konasana, is so named because its movement resembles a butterfly flapping its wings. It targets the legs, offers benefits to the heart and cardiovascular system, relieves anxiety and fatigue, boosts fertility, and dissipates stress. Perform in the morning or evening to relax.

• From a seated position with legs outstretched in a V, bend your knees and brings your calves under your thighs.
• Place your feet together, sole to sole, as close to the pelvis as possible, and clasp your toes with both hands.
• Lower your knees to the floor, pressing gently with elbows if necessary. Inhale deeply and then begin to raise and lower your thighs.
• Continue for 5 to 10 minutes.
Tip: Be sure to sit up straight, with your chin elevated and eyes forward. Don't curl forward.

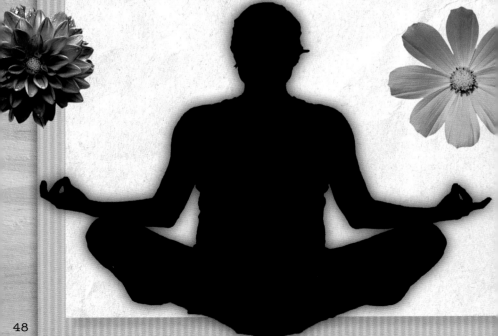

CRESCENT LUNGE

This dynamic standing pose is also known as Anjaneyasana or the High Lunge. In Hindu mythology, it is the pose assumed by monkey god Hanuman of the Ramayana. It stretches and strengthens the lower and upper body and improves stability and balance. It builds mental focus; opens the lungs, chest, and shoulders; invigorates digestion; and increases concentration.

• Begin by standing with your arms at your sides; step the ball of your right foot to the back of the mat. Keep feet slightly apart.
• Pull your abdominals in and up, inhale, then sweep both arms straight overhead with palms facing inward.
• Bend front knee to 90 degrees, keeping knee aligned above ankle. Bend back knee a little and lengthen tailbone toward floor.
• Hold for 5 breaths before switching to opposite legs.
Tip: Press back foot firmly to the floor to aid with balance. Keep hips low and level and facing forward.

LION POSE

Simhasana is known as the "destroyer of all disease." The pose is accompanied by an exaggerated open mouth with the tongue extended down, meant to simulate the lion's roar. The pose removes tension (especially in the face and chest), improves circulation, and keeps bad breath away.

• Kneel down, sitting on your heels, then lean forward onto your spread palms.
• Lower your jaw, open your mouth as wide as possible, and inhale through your nose.
• Stretch your tongue out and curl it down toward your chin.
• Contract the muscles of your throat as you exhale slowly through your mouth with an audible "ha-a-a-a" sound. Gaze upward or focus on the tip of your nose as you roar.
• Hold for as long as is comfortable; repeat often.
Tip: Hands can be kept at sides and swept forward to press the floor as you roar. Also, ankles can be crossed behind you or knees can be widened.

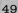

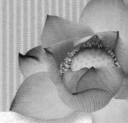

COOL DOWN POSES

CAMEL POSE

This intermediate pose, Ustrasana, is known to open up the entire front of the body, as well as strengthening the spine and stretching the chest, abdominals, hip flexors, thighs, and ankles. In addition to stimulating digestion and the nervous system, it increases blood flow to the face. Avoid if you have high or low blood pressure.

• Kneel with your knees hip-width apart and your tailbone tucked in.
• Place your hands on the back of your waist, fingertips down, and ease your upper torso back. Exhale, and elongate your spine as you press pelvis upward and shoulder blades back.
• Dip slightly to the left and place left hand on left heel. Dip to the right and place right hand on right heel. Arch back, lift chest, drop head back, and relax throat.
• Hold for 20 to 30 seconds; contract stomach, lift chest forward, and raise hands to lower back to release pose.
Tip: Do not compress lower back or rush into the bend. While in pose, center your weight between your knees.

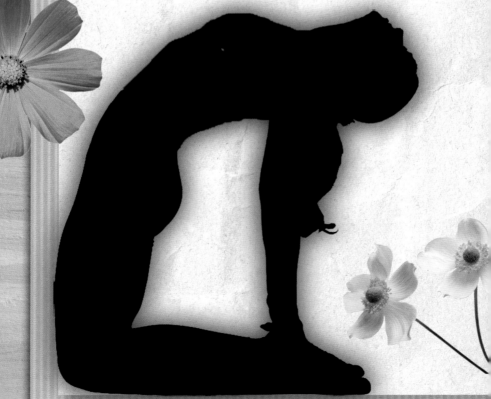

COBRA POSE

Bhujangasana is one of the postures in the Surya Namaskar sun salutation. The name comes from the pose's similarity to the raised hood of a cobra. It opens the chest and benefits the lungs and heart, stimulates the digestive and reproductive systems, eases the symptoms of asthma, and reduces fatigue.

- Lie prone with your flattened palms positioned just below your shoulders; keep arms tucked close.
- As you inhale, raise the upper torso from the floor, pushing down with both hands. Lift from the top of the chest, pushing shoulders down and back and pulling the tailbone toward the pubis.
- Elongate the neck as you gaze slightly upward.
- Hold for 15 to 30 seconds.

Tip: Make sure to use back and chest muscles to create the arch, not just the arms. Bend elbows slightly to keep chest open. Keep hips on or close to floor.

CORPSE POSE

Savasana is typically the final pose in an intense yoga class, allowing you to relax so completely that you are able to switch off both mind and body. Remain in the pose for at least 10 or 12 minutes, but do not fall asleep. You should arise feeling refreshed and renewed. Do not perform if you have a back injury.

THINK ABOUT IT: SHOELESS YOGA
Students often question why it's preferable to go barefoot during yoga sessions. This is because you need to actually feel the mat with your feet as you attempt to balance and stabilize yourself while in certain postures.

- Lie on your back with your arms angled slightly away from your sides.
- Widen shoulders and collarbone so that your arms are positioned with palms face up, fingers in a relaxed curl. Elongate neck but do not tilt head.
- Spread your feet a comfortable distance apart with toes facing outward.
- Close your eyes and relax as you focus on aligning your body and breathing evenly.
- Tune out noises and other distractions.

Tip: Once you feel yourself in alignment, try not to move. You can also try this pose with knees bent and soles flat on the floor.

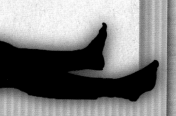

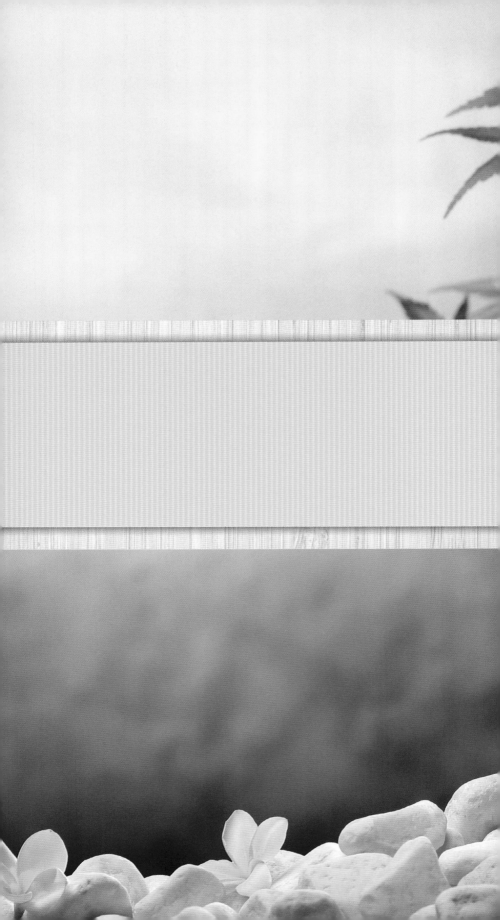

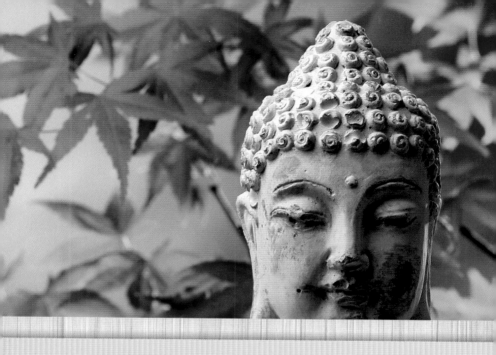
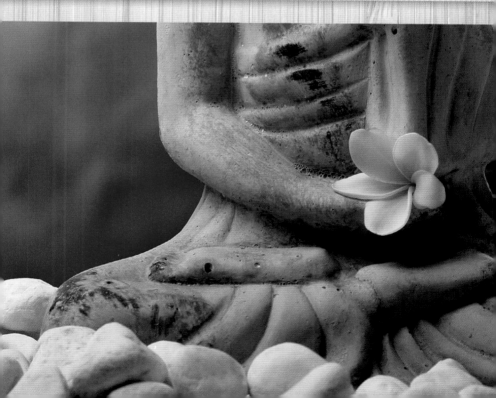

CHAPTER 2

EXPLORING
MEDITATION

EXPLORING MEDITATION

Meditation reached new levels of popularity in the 1960s and 1970s as part of the youth counterculture's quest for enlightenment and self-knowledge. Pop stars meditated and promoted its calming effects, and self-help books lauded its benefits to a generation hooked on tuning in to the zeitgeist and jettisoning mainstream beliefs. Today it is a valued tool for devotees of yoga, Eastern spirituality, and other alternative philosophies.

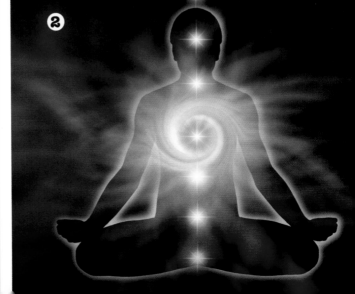

1 Crystal healing
2 Chakra meditation
3 Room for meditation
4 Meditation

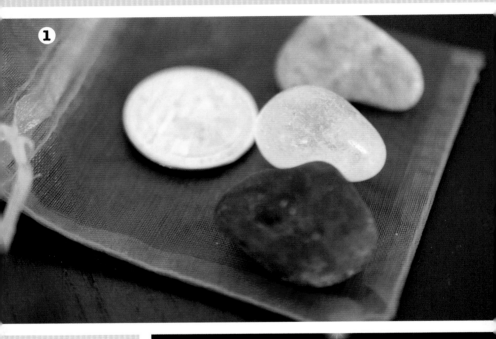

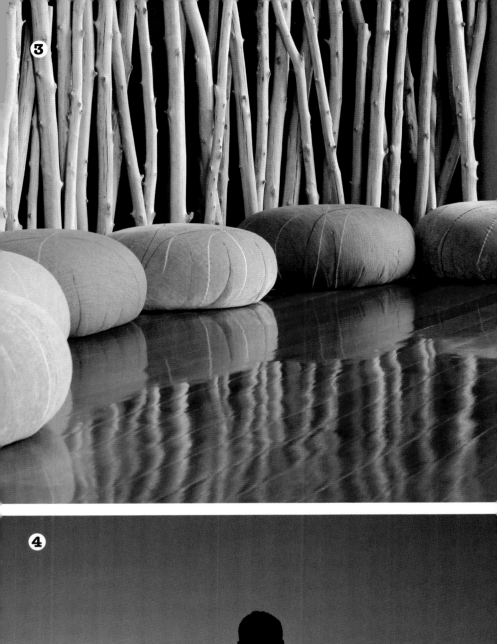

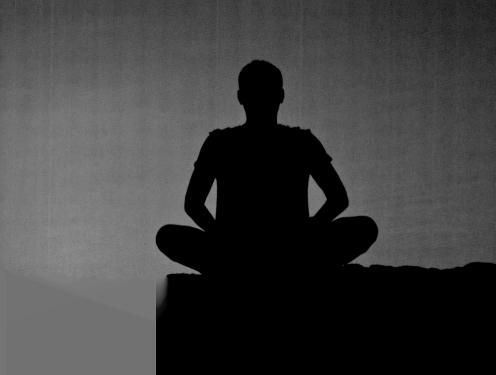

UNDERSTANDING MEDITATION

Meditation is a calm, concentrated inward journey, accompanied by rhythmic breathing, with the goal of achieving a deeper state of consciousness. Individual gains from the practice can vary, but the overall consensus is that it brings peace—and even bliss.

Modern men and women aren't the first to seek respite from unquiet thoughts or ponder the deeper meaning of things. Starting with the philosophers of antiquity, continuing through medieval scribes and Renaissance thinkers, up to our own contemporary authors and scientists, men and woman of introspection and curious natures have always sought answers to life's perplexing questions. And for many of them, these answers were found not by studying the great literature or scientific journals of the day, but by journeying inward to that most "undiscovered country" of all: the human mind.

Aristotle wrote, "Knowing yourself is the beginning of all wisdom." Socrates said, "My friend . . . care for your psyche . . . know thyself, for once we know ourselves, we may learn how to care for ourselves." Poet Alexander Pope said, "Know thyself, presume not God to scan; the proper study of mankind is man." Author Aldous Huxley said, "The more powerful and original a mind, the more it will incline toward the religion of solitude." Elizabeth Gilbert, the author or *Eat, Pray, Love*, reminds us, "Your treasure—your perfection—is within you already. But to claim it, you must leave the busy commotion of the mind, and abandon the desire of the ego, and enter into the silence of the heart."

Each writer is advocating for a form of introspection or self-study that over time has come to fall under the blanket term "meditation." Meditation is a purposeful pursuit that becomes integrated into the lives of practitioners—a valued mental accessory that helps them approach a tumultuous world with balance and serenity. It is not a temporary crutch; it is a continuous bulwark. Furthermore, this activity requires no equipment and little preparation, and can be initiated in almost any quiet spot. And the benefits are manifold: in addition to offering self-knowledge, clarity, and a balm to the spirit, it relieves stress, alters brain-wave patterns, decreases lactic acid in the blood, and lowers oxygen consumption and heart rate.

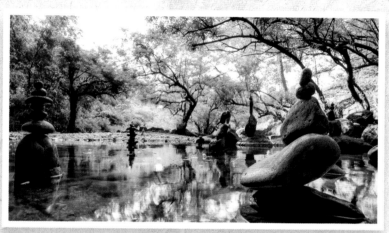

Zen meditation landscape

PRACTICING DHYANA

The act of meditation—or dhyana, in yoga—refers to a precise technique used to rest the mind and attain an elevated state of consciousness unlike the normal waking state. It does not refer to thinking hard about a problem, nor is it daydreaming. Its goal is an understanding of all one's inner levels and ultimately experiencing the highest consciousness possible. Practitioners consider meditation a science, one with distinct principles, with a progression that is to be followed, and with verifiable results.

Meditation can teach you to:
• Cultivate stillness and examine what is within you.
• Calm yourself and let go of your biases.
• Focus fully on one aspect of your body—your muscles, your breathing, or the different levels of your being.
• Train your mind to avoid distractions and resist endless churning.
• Explore your inner dimensions as a means of knowing yourself better.
• Experience your essential nature, which has been described as happiness, peace, and bliss.

The result of successful meditation is frequently a powerful sense of joy and liberation, a gratification that adherents insist is immense and ongoing. As guru H. W. L. Poonja pointed out, "Look within, there is no difference between Yourself, Self, and Guru. You are always Free. There is no teacher, no student, no teaching."

A HISTORY OF MEDITATION

Over the centuries, meditation has been incorporated into a number of religious traditions, including Buddhist, Vedic, Christian, Chinese, and Judaic. Yet the practice is less about belief in a religion or faith than it is about achieving awareness and inner peace.

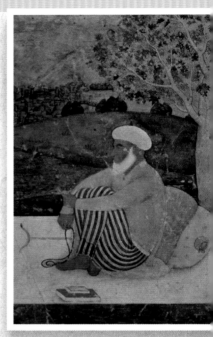

A Sufi saint in Muraqaba meditation, c. 1630

Meditation is an ancient method of transforming the mind that has been practiced in many parts of the world. In primitive cultures, shamans likely entered into a meditative state in order to seek instructions or guidance from the spirit world. Written records that discuss traditions of meditation appear in the Hindu Vedas from around 1500 BC onward, and meditation was likely incorporated into early Hindu teachings. From the sixth to fifth centuries BC, Taoist China and Buddhist India began developing their own forms of meditation.

In the Mediterranean region, around 20 BC, Philo of Alexandria wrote of "spiritual exercises" involving deep concentration, and Greek philosopher Plotinus experimented with meditative techniques in the third century. Saint Augustine investigated the Greek's methods but "did not achieve ecstasy." Later, the advent of the mercantile Silk Road to Asia spread aspects of Buddhism to other countries, including the concept of Zen meditation to China. Judaism may have been bequeathed its meditative practices from earlier Israeli traditions, or they might have existed from the start. In Genesis, Isaac was said to go into "lasuach"—a meditative trance.

In eigth-century Japan, Buddhism began to increase in earnest, and meditative practices brought from China by the monk Dosho in 653 were further developed. As more practices arrived from China, they continued to be modified and refined. In 1227, when the monk Dogen returned from China with the written steps for *zazen*, or sitting meditation, a community of meditative Zen monks was conceived.

CHRISTIAN MEDITATION

In eastern Europe during the Byzantine period, between the tenth and fourteenth centuries, a tradition of contemplation called hesychasm developed. It required the repetition of the Jesus prayer, and may have been influenced by Indian or Sufi mystics. Christian meditation of western Europe tended not to use repetition or require specific postures. In the 1500s, the practice was further modified by saints such as Ignatius of Loyola and Teresa of Avila.

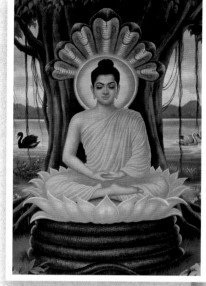

Buddha protected by a seven-headed cobra

MODERN MEDITATION

During the eighteenth century, European intellectuals had a penchant for "Orientalism" in general and the study of Buddhism in particular. German philosopher Schopenhauer discussed it in salons and the French writer Voltaire begged tolerance for Buddhists. The first English translation of the Tibetan Book of the Dead appeared in 1927. Swami Vivekananda had already aroused Western interest in yoga and meditation, and subsequent visiting gurus kept interest in Indian mysticism keen. Secular schools of yoga and meditation meant for non-Hindus began to evolve, focusing more on stress reduction, relaxation, and self-improvement than on spiritual awakening. Among these were forms of hatha yoga and of transcendental meditation (TM), which became popular in the 1960s when the Beatles visited its creator, Maharishi Mahesh Yogi.

Not surprisingly, both the spiritual and secular types of meditation became subjects of scientific testing in the 1950s. Yet after more than six decades of analysis, the mechanisms of meditation have continued to elude scientists.

WHAT'S IT MEAN? JUBU.

This terms refers to Jewish Buddhists who practice Buddhist-based meditation for spiritual, but not necessarily religious, purposes. They have become an influence on current Western attitudes toward meditation. The group, which reflects an explosion of interest within the Jewish community, has included many luminaries, including Leonard Cohen, Robert Downey Jr., Allen Ginsberg, Philip Glass, Mandy Patinkin, and Goldie Hawn.

CHOOSING A DISCIPLINE

Whether you are looking to reduce stress, increase self-awareness, create a spiritual connection, achieve stillness, or gain enlightenment through movement, some form of meditation is sure to offer the results you are seeking.

Currently the six most popular categories of meditation are mindfulness, spiritual, focused, movement, mantra, and transcendental. As with any new interest, you may need to try several variations before you find the one that best suits your needs.

Mindfulness: This method, which combines concentration with awareness, is intended to steady the mind, clarify thoughts, and reduce stress. It is based on Buddhist teachings and is now the most popular form of meditation in the West. As you meditate, you pay attention to thoughts or feelings that pass through your mind, but you do not become involved in them. You can focus on breathing or on an object. Mindfulness is ideal for those who want to meditate alone.

Spiritual: This form of meditation is associated with Eastern religions such as Hinduism and Daoism and also with Christianity. It replicates silent prayer as you seek a deeper connection with your god or the universe. Essential oils such as frankincense, myrrh, sage, and cedar can enhance the experience. It can be practiced in the home or in a place or worship.

Focused: This method involves concentration using one of the five senses—for instance, focusing on breathing, counting mala beads, inhaling a calming scent, gazing at a candle, or listening to soothing chimes. Although it sounds simple, this form of meditation can be difficult—many students have trouble maintaining focus for any length of time.

Movement: In addition to yoga poses, this practice can involve walking in the woods, gardening, qigong, or any other gentle type of motion. The movement actually guides you into a meditative state, and it is a good choice for students who like to let their minds wander.

Mantra: This form of meditation occurs in many teachings, especially Hindu and Buddhist. It uses a repetitive word or sound, which can be chanted softly or loudly, to clear the mind. As you chant, you will find yourself in tune with your environment and able to seek deeper levels of consciousness. The mantra also allows students to focus on sound rather than breathing.

Transcendental: This is the most popular form of meditation in the world. It is also the most scientifically studied. Although it uses a mantra, each mantra is specific to the individual student. It is a pursuit that offers structure but requires serious dedication.

DIY: Black Out

A visualization exercise called palming is an easy way to lower stress. Simply cover your closed eyes with your hands and concentrate on the color black, filling your entire visual field with the color. Or focus on a color you associate with anxiety, like bright red or orange, and then replace it with a color that makes you feel calm and safe.

OTHER THERAPEUTIC METHODS

Traditional meditation is not the only way to commune with the inner self. These other methods can have an effect similar to meditation and offer a number of the same restorative benefits

Biofeedback: In this mind-body technique, individuals monitor body parts electronically and learn to modify their physiology in order to improve their physical, mental, emotional, and spiritual state. This technique has been used to address back pain, headaches, anxiety disorders, and muscle retraining after injury or surgery.

Visualization: Humans are naturally prone to daydreaming and creating imaginary scenarios—examples of the visualization process. Scientists have discovered that by visualizing certain feats—say, hitting a baseball or passing an exam—an individual may come closer to achieving them. This technique, which is popular with athletes, can also be used as a relaxation or therapeutic tool to combat depression or anxiety.

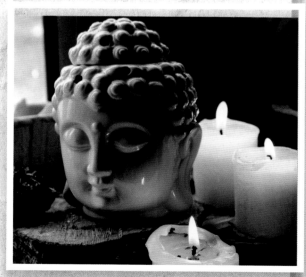

Face of Buddha

SOUND AND VIBRATION

Sound or vibration can be a factor in several types of meditation, and singing bowls, gongs, drumming, or soft music certainly help to facilitate the experience. But perhaps the most important sound is that of your own voice chanting a personal mantra.

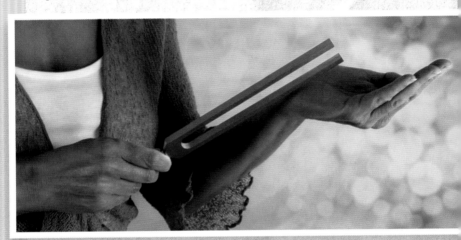

Sound healer with tuning fork

Sound therapy is based on the premise that all types of matter, including the cells in our bodies, vibrate at different frequencies. These vibrations can be optimized to combat stress, emotional woes, and disease.

Many students learn to practice meditation with a mantra. This consists of a sound, vibration, word, or group of words that is repeated as a point of focus to help the student enter a state of profound relaxation. In Sanskrit, *mantra* translates as "vehicle of the mind," which it certainly can be. People may speak their mantra aloud, whisper it, or intone it silently. Some students do not speak their mantra in the presence of others; they believe it is theirs alone. Many practitioners simply stick with the universal "om" or "aum," which is considered the first sound of creation. Or they find a phrase in Sanskrit that appeals to them, such as *om mani podme hum*, which translates loosely to "the jewel in the lotus flower."

LISTEN AND LEARN

There are several types of meditation that use sound or vibration as their focus rather than breathing.

Music Meditation: This is probably the most mainstream form of sound therapy, and many music therapists have board certification. It is used to relieve pain, loneliness, and depression, and is often provided in clinics, hospitals, and hospices.

Sound Meditation: This popular practice incorporates traditional Tibetan instruments, such as singing bowls, to help clear the mind and allow the student to enter a deep state of quiet awareness.

Gong Therapy: This is like sound meditation in the extreme—the participants lie on a mat with a blanket and pillow and are "bathed" in healing gong sound waves. The instructor guides the meditation, playing the gong softly at first, but increasing the volume as the session progresses. To avoid a monotonous rhythm, the sound of the gong changes frequently. This auditory stimulus leads to what is known as entrainment, a form of beneficially modified brain-wave frequencies. The first state to be reached is alpha, which lies between eight and twelve Hz. This is a relaxed creative state associated with daydreams and imaginative thinking. Next comes an influx of theta waves, which fall between four and seven Hz and are associated with deep meditation, REM sleep, and hypnosis.

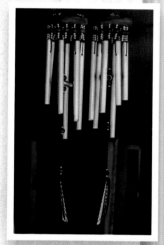

Gong therapy dates back thousands of years and is an important part of healing kundalini meditation. It is employed to reduce stress, open emotional blockages, promote vitality, and increase happiness; there are even scientific indications that certain types of sound therapy encourage damaged DNA strands to repair themselves.

Wind chimes

Primordial Sound Meditation: This powerful form of medication is rooted in the Vedic traditions of India and is about "restful awareness," making your inner silence part of your life. This discipline utilizes a personal mantra that is calculated mathematically based on the vibrations created by the universe at your time and place of birth; this mantra is repeated silently, never aloud.

FEEL THE VIBES

It might be hard for many Westerners—and a few Easterners—to comprehend that a meditating body can physically vibrate. Yet quite a number of practitioners have experienced this, a rhythmic shaking throughout their torso and limbs, especially during a long or intense session. This may be due to pent-up negative energies finally being expelled, in a sort of psychic/psychological cleansing.

LEARNING TO CHANNEL INWARD

It may be a case of "easier said than done": many meditation students discover that finding stillness or quieting the mind is no simple task. Yet there are proven steps for transcending all the external noise and emotional distractions and truly turning inward.

THE FOUR ELEMENTS

Systems of meditation may differ, but most require four basic elements: a quiet space, a formal posture, an object to focus on, and a passive, receptive attitude.

1. The main requisite for successful meditation is learning to be still. This begins with finding a quiet, relaxing space in which to practice.

2. The second requirement is a posture that allows you to be erect, comfortable, and alert. In yoga, the student is taught to keep the head, neck, and trunk aligned while sitting in a meditative pose, or asana. Once you have mastered a suitable meditative pose, you should always use the same posture. It also helps to meditate at the same time and in the same place each day. Some students wear a light shawl when they meditate, believing that the shawl replicates the vibrations from the previous day's meditation.

Begin by sitting in a firm chair or on a comfortable pillow with your back upright and your eyes closed. Focus on each part of your body, allowing all the muscles to relax except in the neck and back. Take your time, reveling in the feeling of letting go. As your body gives in to this liberating sensation, your mind will soon follow. Next focus on your breathing: become aware of how your lungs draw air in and then expel it. To truly relax, lower your breathing from your chest to your diaphragm; observe your breathing but do not control it.

3. As you attempt to "keep your thoughts in the present moment," begin focusing on an object, a sound, or a word. Some Buddhist monks focus on an unanswerable question, or koan; these can free you from the limits of rational thought.

4. Your restless mind will likely supply many worrisome thoughts, but do not heed them. Let your mind wander before bringing it back into focus. This is the trick, many students say, of successful meditation. Hear the thoughts but do not react to them—it is not the thoughts but your reaction to them that distracts you. This is the beginning of understanding the person you can be without all that mental churning.

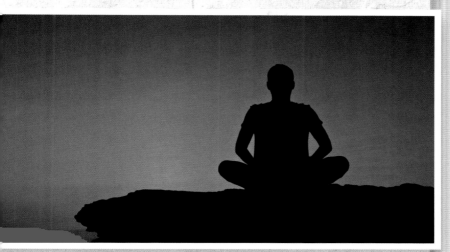

Meditation instills deeper levels of relaxation or calmness

CHOOSING YOUR REACTION

Conversely, by practicing meditation and not reacting to random thoughts while in that state, you will now be open and attentive to any problems or questions that come before you in daily life. The uncertainty, anger, moodiness, depression, or other heightened emotions you typically feel when something negative happens will no longer goad you. Now, you will face discord with a sense of awareness, for instance: "I am feeling very threatened by this encounter." The emotion will be experienced, it will move through you, and you will then have a range of calmer emotions to choose from before deciding how to address the problem. In other words, you won't be the victim of your volatile emotions: you will observe them, and then choose an alternative reaction—rationality, serenity, enthusiasm, determination, humor—that is best suited to the situation.

Meditation also strips off some of the masks people wear; it reveals inner complexes, immature behaviors, and unproductive habits. Again, you will now be able to give these issues your full attention, coming up with strategies to weed them out of your life. This is the only way in which such things ever really clear—by examining them in the light of day.

The beneficial effects of meditation may occur slowly, over a period of time. There may be no dramatic "Eureka!" moment. You will probably notice small things at first—deeper levels of relaxation or calmness. You may realize that you fret less over problems. If you continue with your practice, eventually you will feel free of the commonplace worries that trouble most of us. And that is a good indicator that soon you will be able to be fully present and fully receptive as you enter the meditative state.

BALANCING YOUR CHAKRAS

To improve your chi, or life force, you must balance the seven key points where energy flows through the body. These are the *chakras*—Sanskrit for "wheels of light"—or energy portals that interact with both the body and the spirit.

Many students of spiritual practices and philosophies believe that humans possess an energy field that radiates a few feet from their bodies. When energy passes from this field into the body, it is transformed by the centers of spiritual power, the chakras, into thought, emotion, and physical sensation. Just as the brain interprets the different frequencies of light that enter the eyes as colors, so the chakras interpret the frequencies and vibrations of energy and form the impressions that impact us.

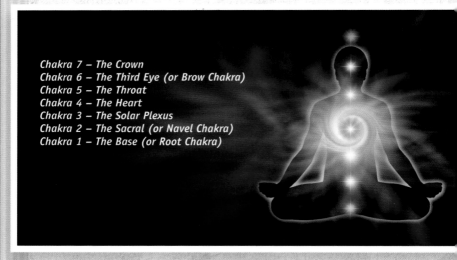

Chakra 7 – The Crown
Chakra 6 – The Third Eye (or Brow Chakra)
Chakra 5 – The Throat
Chakra 4 – The Heart
Chakra 3 – The Solar Plexus
Chakra 2 – The Sacral (or Navel Chakra)
Chakra 1 – The Base (or Root Chakra)

The seven chakras

The seven chakras are located along the central meridian of the body. Each is associated with a certain body part, color, and domain.

1. The first or root chakra, Muladhara, is located at the base of the spine, or coccyx, and is represented by the color red. It governs the understanding of the physical dimension.

2. Second, Svadhishthana, is the sacral chakra, located just above the genitals. It is associated with the color orange and regulates sexual energy.

3. The third, Manipura, is the solar plexus chakra; it is designated by the color yellow and controls creative power.

4. The heart chakra, Anahata, is fourth, and is represented as emerald green. It controls circulation and breathing.

5. Fifth is the blue throat chakra, Vishuddha, which represents the intellectual body, personal integrity, and identity.

6. Sixth is the third eye or face chakra, Ajna, located on the forehead and shown as deep indigo. It controls all thoughts and visions.

7. The seventh chakra, Sahasrara, is the highest chakra in terms of frequency. It is known as the crown chakra and it synchronizes all colors and manifests as white light. It controls the upper brain, the nervous system, and the pineal gland, and is associated with spirituality.

CHAKRA MEDITATION

The relaxation techniques that bring balance and well-being to the chakras are quite basic. You can focus one, several, or all seven chakras in turn. Start by sitting erect in a comfortable chair. Close your eyes, and begin belly breathing. Concentrate on the first chakra at the base of your spine, home to dormant kundalini energy. Imagine you are breathing in and out through this chakra, visualizing it as a fiery red ball. Allow your consciousness to sink into and become the ball, and feel it being drawn downward to the earth. Pay attention to how you are feeling physically, emotionally, and mentally. Remain in this state for eight to 10 minutes, and tell yourself, "Whenever I reach this relaxed state I will learn to use my mind more creatively and become aware of the energy blocks that have impeded me."

Afterward, release the ball of energy, slowly count to five, and open your eyes. You should feel refreshed and peaceful. You can stop there or work your way up, making sure to give each chakra its proper color and attribute as you visualize it.

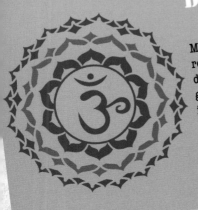

DIY: Cherish the Crown

Meditating to repair the crown chakra can remove blockages that are making you depressed, sluggish, frustrated, or even greedy. A restored crown will bring you insight, mindfulness, and self-confidence. Yoga, crystal therapy, and aromatherapy are also beneficial for this powerful chakra, which offers the potential for universal connection.

THE ART OF RELAXATION

Medical researchers now know that relaxing is not just a pleasant pastime reserved for weekend afternoons, but rather a daily necessity that promotes mental and physical well-being. Even if you never master meditation, you can certainly learn to relax.

Doctors are quick to tell harried or anxious patients that they need to relax more, but few ever spell out the steps that such a lifestyle adjustment requires. If all it took to shake off tension was a walk in the park or a few yoga classes, many fewer people would be suffering the debilitating effects of stress—including high blood pressure, tension headaches, backaches, obesity, addiction, depression, and anxiety. And although there are medications that can help people manage stress, why not start by addressing the situation in a more natural manner?

The good news is that there are relaxing behaviors you can learn that, though lacking the deeply soothing effects of meditation, can still allow you to calm down and stop fretting. And even if you are accomplished at meditation, there are situations where it is not practical—in an office cubicle or on a crowded train—where you should opt for relaxation therapy.

SLOWING DOWN

Below are some useful tips for taking the edge off your frazzled nerves:

• Even if you don't meditate, you can borrow some techniques. Sit erect in a comfortable chair and focus on your breathing, keeping it even and unhurried. Ease into progressive muscle relaxing—starting with your toes, tense them for 5 seconds, relax them for thirty, and repeat several times. Work up from there to your head and neck, addressing all the muscle groups along the way.

• Use your evening commuter time to decompress by listening to soothing music, calling an old friend, or opening a free meditation app like Insight Timer, Calm, or Stop, Breathe, and Think to ease you out of that "rat-race" mentality.

- Log off from social media for a night or two. The American Psychological Association reports that the more a person checks their Twitter or Facebook accounts, the higher their level of stress. Women are particularly vulnerable. Let these websites and apps exist without your input for a time, and you'll come back to them in better fettle.

- Likewise, unplug from electronic devices on which you feel dependent. Read a book, visit with a friend, or simply go for a drive and enjoy the scenery instead.

- A lot of our tension builds up at work, and especially affects our back and shoulders, so it helps to loosen them during the day. While seated at your desk, interlock your curled fingers and perform 10 isometric pulls, alternating five seconds tense, 10 seconds relaxed. Then place your palms together and do isometric pushes. Raise both arms over your head and push up against an imaginary barrier for a five count. Then push out to the side with both arms.

- Stop making multiple lists, memos, and sticky note reminders of the many things you still need to do. These little "nudgers" can make your life feel out of control. Instead, prepare one list, hang it in plain sight, and check off each task as you complete it.

- Prioritize your "to-do" list and place people-related activities above cleaning, clearing, and decluttering. That is not to say you should ignore your weekly chores, but human interactions are more effective at reducing stress than a weekend spent redoing your closet.

- How often is it that you feel as though your free time is eaten up by minutia? Make a list of the activities you love, the ones that leave you mellow or fulfilled, and assign yourself one of them the next time you have an open afternoon. Hit that vintage book barn in the country or take the family to the science museum, or do whatever other activity brings you joy.

- Become so immersed in whatever you are doing that you feel connected to it in a healthy way—whether you're wandering in nature, coloring in pictures of mandalas, or taking a cooking class—and try to discover new aspects of each pastime.

- Don't be afraid to say no to activities that are supposed to relax you but that you yourself don't enjoy. Things such as gardening, massage, shopping, salon visits, reading the newspaper, or breakfast in bed can actually raise stress levels in many people.

PREPARE A MEDITATION SPACE

Nothing is more conducive to home meditation than having a dedicated space in which to practice. Surround yourself with familiar objects and soothing sounds, as well as inspirational photos or artwork, anything that reminds you to stay calm and focused.

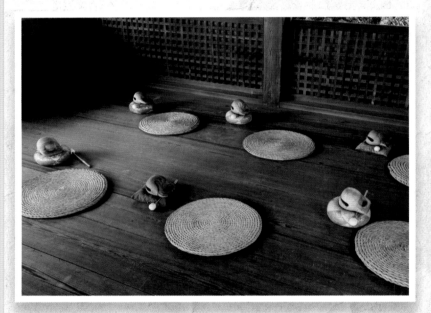

Although it's true that it takes little preparation or equipment to meditate, it makes sense to have your own designated space at home, especially if you are just starting out and require solitude. The main stipulation is that it be somewhere quiet, where you can remain undisturbed for half an hour or so—a corner of a bedroom, a small studio, an insulated sunporch, even a roomy closet. It is a plus if you have a window with natural light; otherwise the interior lighting should not be harsh. A few small table lamps with soft-light bulbs will do fine. Make sure there is something to focus on, such as a tropical fish tank, a group of plants, or a collection of flameless candles.

Soft surfaces are also key. Place a plush area rug on the floor along with several large pillows or cushions for seating. If you prefer to meditate sitting upright in a chair, make sure it is comfortable and supportive. Or consider a round, padded ottoman.

MEANINGFUL OBJECTS

Although the decor of your space should reflect simplicity, there are certain items that may help you become more receptive to the process.

• Inspirational artwork and statuary will remind students of their connection to the divine, or their higher power. Many people include the Buddha in one of his numerous poses or postures—laughing, touching earth, reclining, and so on—or one of the Hindu deities.

• Many practitioners find that music helps them to journey inward, so consider adding a small CD or MP3 player. Some claim the soothing sounds of a small fountain can help them relax. Others use singing bowls or the clicking of meditation beads, called japamala, to aid them.

• The smell of incense has long been associated with spiritual connection. Try sampling scents like healing sandalwood, the favorite of Buddhist temples; mood-elevating jasmine; stress-easing lavender; cleansing pine or cedar; relaxing chamomile; or restorative lemongrass.

• In one corner tuck a small bookcase or shelf for your related books and DVDs. Even masters of meditation remain lifelong students as they continue to learn new paths.

• Some parents invite their children into the space—as a quiet place to relax or to practice mindful breathing with mom or dad. Children enjoy creating "mind jars," mason jars filled with water, glitter, and small shells or colored stones. They shake the jar and then focus on mindful breathing as they watch the glitter swirl.

DIY: Create a Meditation Altar

Many practitioners find a small altar makes an ideal point of concentration. Cover a low table or bench with a decorative scarf or piece of fabric. Then add a photo, image, or statue of an inspirational icon—Christ, Buddha, or perhaps one of the gurus you have read about in your meditation studies—and surround it with candles and meaningful objects. Add fresh flowers or garlands as tributes. The altar should be pleasing to both the eye and spirit.

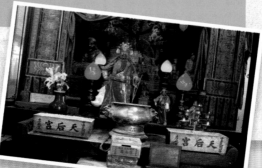

Shrine and altar in the Buddhist Tin Hau temple, Hong Kong

OVERCOMING ADDICTION

In recent years meditation has been used effectively to help people quit smoking and control overeating. It is now being used to help alcoholics and drug addicts overcome their addictions, maintain sobriety, and remain in recovery.

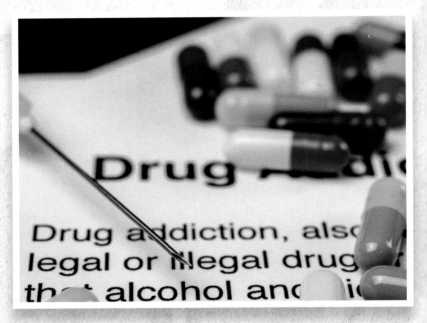

By now everyone knows that smoking is one of the unhealthiest habits a person can cultivate. It not only causes respiratory diseases and lung cancer, but the toxins in cigarettes infiltrate and damage nearly every organ in the body and compromise circulation. Smoking shortens the lifespan and impacts quality of life. Yet cigarettes are one of the most difficult substances to permanently withdraw from—according to researchers, nicotine may be as addictive as hard drugs such as heroin.

There is new help, however, for those who have been unable to quit while using medications or going cold turkey. Recent studies report that mindfulness-type meditation offers both mental and physical support to those who want to quit, and it further increases their chances of success. Meditation has also worked for chronic overeaters who are trying to cut down consumption. There are many guided meditations available on the internet that can assist novices to reach deeper levels of consciousness in order to break bad or destructive habits.

Below are some of the ways that meditation can help smokers "banish the butts."

• Meditation reduces stress, which is often a trigger for smokers. They believe that smoking relaxes them and eases tension, but the truth is that cigarettes simply mask the stress—and increase heart rate. With meditation, the smoker soon understands what is causing the stress and can find ways, besides smoking, of controlling it.

• Meditating can make people aware of their cravings and then help reduce them. Through meditation, the smoker mindfully experiences their physical and mental states, such as the cravings and edginess that occur when cigarettes are withheld. Once these factors are recognized, the smoker can begin to accept the feelings and start to reshape their own behavior.

• People who smoke often lament that they have no self-control when it comes to quitting. The good news is that research on subjects who meditate regularly has shown enhanced connectivity in the regions of the brain that are linked to self-control. Don't be surprised if meditating suddenly gives you the willpower to stop smoking or to stop snacking before bedtime. In fact, some smokers report that they started curbing their habit without even realizing it.

BEYOND 12 STEPS

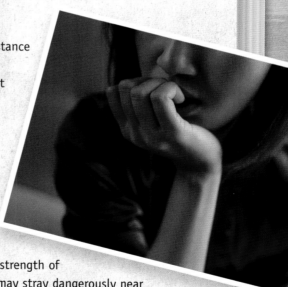

The appeal of any addictive substance or activity—narcotics, alcohol, gambling, shopping, sex—is that it furnishes an intense high, a feeling of euphoria on which the user becomes hooked. Even cigarette smokers report the pleasurable rush of that first inhalation of the morning. But as their tolerance increases, the highs become harder to achieve; the abuser has to increase frequency of use or the strength of the substance. As a result, they may stray dangerously near toxic intake levels of alcohol or drugs in order to find satisfaction. This is why "kicking the habit" is so crucial—it saves lives.

There are a number of systems available for treating addicts, including the highly successful 12-step program advocated by Alcoholics Anonymous. Mindfulness meditation is just beginning to take its place as another beneficial practice that can break the patterns of addiction. As mentioned above, meditation facilitates self-awareness

OVERCOMING ADDICTION

and enhances self-control; it also allows people to substitute a natural high—and one that is not habit forming—for an artificial one.

Addiction often arises from emotional factors: anxiety, depression, or fear that can make a person succumb to self-destructive behaviors. Some psychologists refer to addicts as having a "wanting mind"—a state of unhappiness that mistakenly depends on material things to alleviate it. Again, meditation can help to fill that desperate "hole in the soul" that addicts know too well and provide a more lasting state of pleasure and fulfillment.

Another core belief of 12-step recovery is faith in a higher power; this can be God or another entity of a person's own choosing. For many centuries meditation has served as a conduit between practitioners and their deities or higher powers, and there are likely few things so encouraging, so reassuring, to someone in addiction recovery as

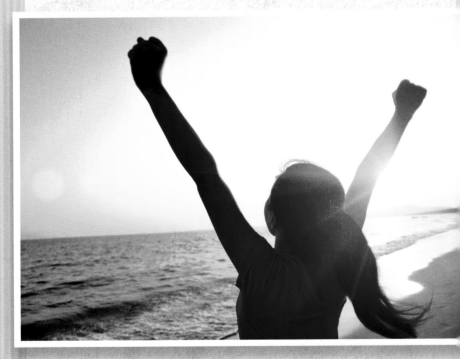

experiencing that satisfying communion with the "godhead" during deep meditation.

Ideally, the optimal course for a recovering addict is a combination of aids: enlisting in a 12-step or other recovery program and augmenting it with meditation therapy at home.

PRACTICING MINDFULNESS

If you are interested in cutting back on cigarettes or food consumption, or if you have a more serious addiction, it is not difficult to master several of the breathing techniques used in mindfulness meditation. The examples below vary in length and purpose.

1. One-Minute Meditation: This exercise stimulates the parasympathetic nervous system, the relaxation response. Sit with your eyes closed and hold a deep breath for a count of four. Exhale for an eight count as you visualize oxygen moving through your bloodstream and your stress floating away.

2. Seven-Minute Meditation: According to a research team at Harvard, this exercise soon develops focus, attention, and a sense of clarity and calm when practiced twice a day. Sit relaxed and erect and take several long, rolling breaths. Begin counting one inhale, one exhale, until you reach 10. Then count again backwards. Repeat the cycle five times, then continue breathing at this steady pace for another few minutes while visualizing the breath moving through your lungs.

3. Five-Minute Body Scan Mediation: This exercise allows you to discover unconscious areas of tension and release them. Studies show this meditation can improve sleep patterns and alleviate fatigue and depression. Sit or lie down in a comfortable pose and ease into a calm, steady breathing pattern. Then focus your awareness on different parts of the body, starting with the left toes. When you find tension, breathe into it and relax it on the exhale. Do the left and right sides first, and then move up to the neck and head.

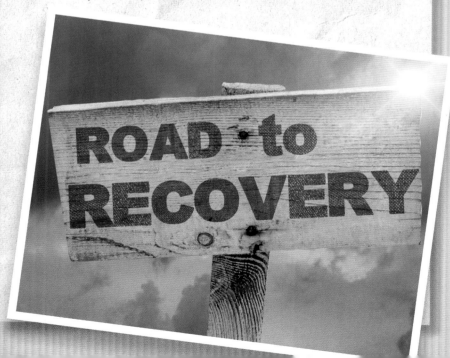

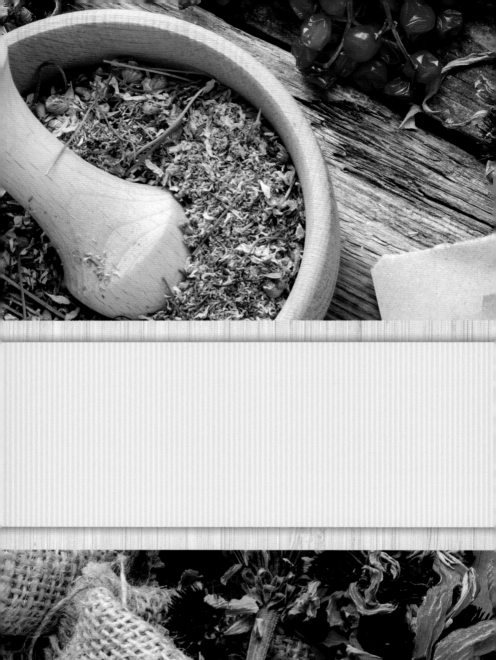

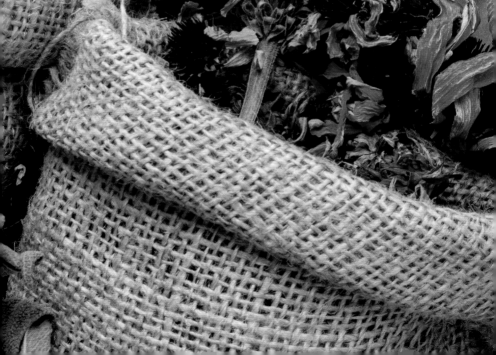

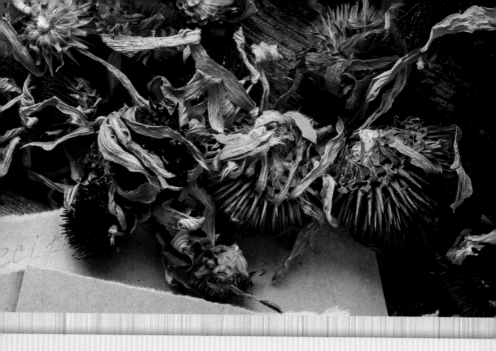

CHAPTER 3
HERBAL REMEDIES

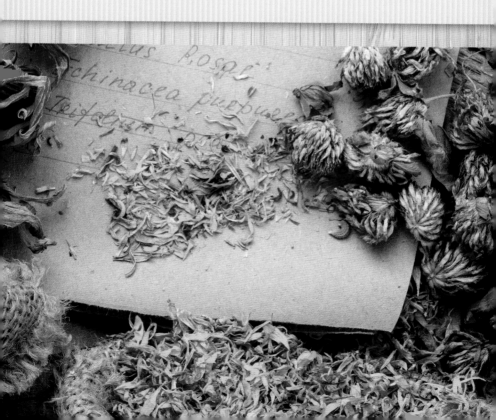

HERBAL REMEDIES AND ESSENTIAL OILS

Before commercial pharmaceuticals existed as big business, even before the dawn of patent medicines—"cures" concocted by doctors or chemists or even quacks—there existed an agrarian culture that went back thousands of years, one that used time-tested herbs and other healing plants to combat sickness and disease, treat wounds and infections, and help ease pregnancy and childbirth.

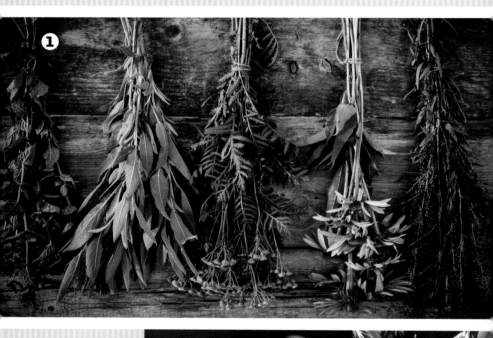

1 Dried herbs
2 Hibiscus
3 Valerian
4 Spikenard
5 Cinnamon tea
6 Garlic and onions

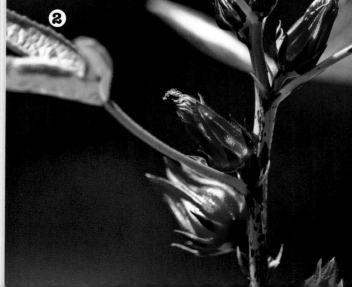

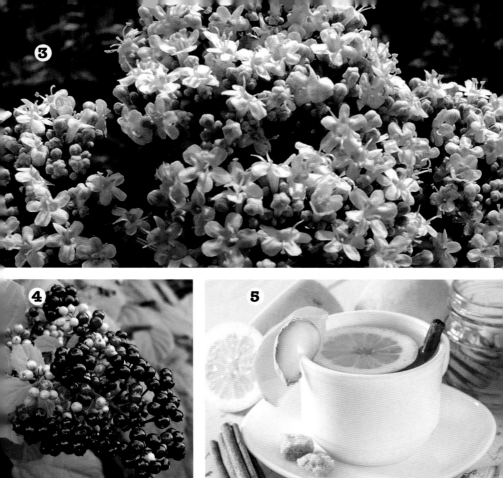

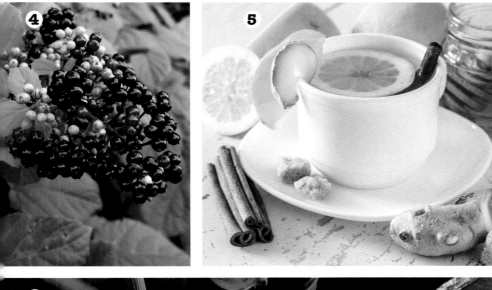

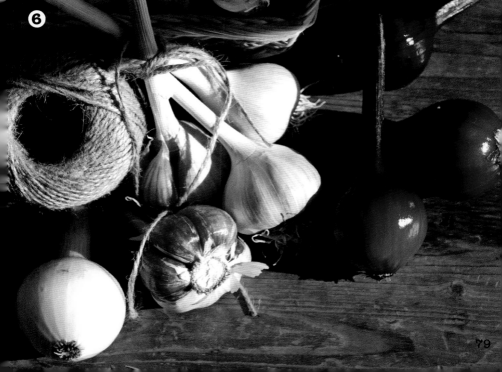

A HISTORY OF HERBAL MEDICINES

Versatile herbs not only offer culinary flavors and mood-elevating scents, they also provide a form of healing called phytomedicine, which dates back to ancient eras and has recently been revisited by the scientific and natural-health communities.

Herbs are generally defined as plants with leaves, seeds, or flowers that are used to flavor food, provide scent, and treat disease. Some or all parts of the plant may be utilized—root, stem, leaf, flower, fruits, and seeds. Essential oils can also be distilled from these plants; they contain concentrations of beneficial compounds as well as vitamins and minerals.

From the earliest established communities of humans, herbs were valued for their ability to combat disease and treat injuries. According to fossil records, ginkgo biloba dates back to the Paleozoic period—and was undoubtedly a curative used by early Homo sapiens. Herbal remedies were eventually found in most ancient cultures: they were praised by the Greeks and Romans, written down in Indian holy books by ayurvedic physicians, utilized throughout the Middle East, detailed in the journals of Chinese doctors, and valued by indigenous people everywhere for use in their healing rituals. But with the advent of modern medicine, sophisticated new drugs nearly supplanted the time-honored herbal remedies. Almost everyone worshipped at the altar of the pharmaceutical. That is, until it turned out that certain serious diseases continued to evade the search for cures, in spite of all the medical advancements. Herbs again came into the spotlight, and went under the microscope. They now offer possibilities for treating, slowing, or even preventing, modern scourges such as cancer, Alzheimer's disease, diabetes, and HIV/AIDS.

SPICES FOR LIFE

Another form of healing botanicals are the spices—food additives typically made from the dried leaves, stems, blooms, seeds, roots, bark, or other parts of plants. Spices originally provided strong flavorings in dishes and helped to prevent food spoilage. Their role was expanded once early healers realized that these seasonings—rich in antioxidants and anti-inflammatories—also had curative effects on the body, mind, and spirit. They were soon being used to treat systemic diseases and infections; pain, joint, and muscle complaints; reproductive issues; anxiety and depression; wounds; and injuries.

By the early Middle Ages, numerous spices were in such demand they became high-value items of barter, some worth their weight in gold. Caravans of Arab traders that carried these treasures and other rarities to the West created the Silk Road, made up of routes to the East that still exist today. Modern transportation means that few spices are so scarce, but they are still prized as culinary flourishes. And when a natural health revival occurred in the 1960s, medicinal spices again came to the fore, especially once scientific research vindicated many of them as genuine remedies and experts began to further understand their beneficial chemistry.

If natural methods of improving or maintaining your health are part of your personal agenda, read on to uncover the surprising world of medicinal herbs and spices.

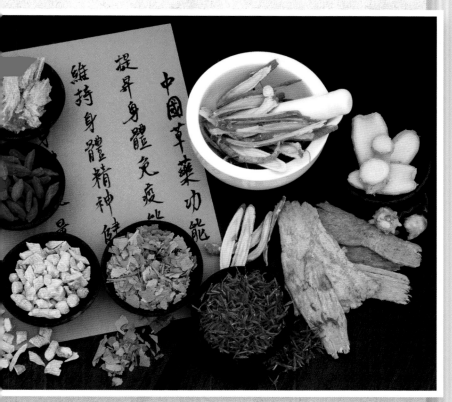

Chinese herbal medicine selection

CULINARY HERBS

Many culinary herbs also have a long, respected history as healing or medicinal herbs. Not only does ingesting them—both in food dishes and in prescribed remedies—bolster health, some can also be applied topically for pain and swelling.

BASIL

A mainstay of Mediterranean cuisine, basil (*Ocimum basilicum*) has earned the title the "king of herbs," and its earthy, spicy-sweet flavor is today found in kitchens worldwide. It can be eaten raw, cooked, sautéed, blended into pesto, and used to make sauces, soups, and salads. This annual member of the mint family, with its spikes of small pale flowers, originated in India, Africa, and Asia. It is effective for treating stomach irritations, nausea, and flatulence. It acts as an appetite enhancer, increases the flow of bile, and helps to clear nasal passages of mucous and harmful bacteria. Dried basil provides calcium, magnesium, and iron.

Basil

BAY LEAF

Bay leaves, either fresh or dried, are added to soups, stews, tomato sauces, and casseroles to provide an earthy flavor. The elliptical glossy green leaves grow on the evergreen bay laurel tree (*Lauris nobilis*), which also produces clusters of yellow or greenish-white star-shaped flowers. The tree, native to Asia Minor, is now found throughout the Mediterranean. The leaves are rich in immunity-boosting vitamin C, antioxidant vitamin A, folic acid, B complex, potassium, calcium, manganese, copper, and selenium. Natural healers used bay to cure stomach ulcers and flatulence. The essential oil can treat arthritis, reduce congestion, and help the body process insulin, thus lowering blood sugar.

Bay leaves

BORAGE

Borago officinalis is native to the Mediterranean, but it is now found worldwide. The plant can reach a height of three feet and features hairy, wrinkled leaves with blue, star-shaped flowers with black anthers. Besides its culinary uses, borage is raised as an agricultural crop—its oil-rich seeds are high in nutrients, and it is the world's leading source of beneficial gamma-linolenic acid (GLA). Natural healers recommend borage to treat diabetes, stress, and high blood pressure, and to decrease inflammation, ease pain, protect the heart, ensure female health, treat skin disorders, aid with weight loss, and calm hyperactivity. Its mucilage content helps ease respiratory problems. The essential oil of borage is often called starflower.

CHERVIL

Medical use of the delicate culinary herb chervil (*Anthriscus cerefolium*) dates to ancient Rome, where it was valued as a diuretic. The medium-sized plant, which originated in the Caucasus Mountains, has curly leaves and small white flowers that form umbels. The herb is an excellent source of antioxidants, which help to stabilize cell membranes and reduce inflammation. It is recommended as an eyewash and as a tea to ease menstrual cramps. Crumpled leaves can be placed on wounds, insect bites, or burns to speed healing; a warm poultice of chervil can ease joints swollen by arthritis or injury.

Chervil

CHIVES

Mild-flavored chives (*Allium schoenoprasum*) are the smallest members of the onion family, with thin, hollow, edible stems. They are native to North America, Europe, and parts of Asia. Health-wise, they can lower LDL bad cholesterol and improve heart health, and their high levels of vitamin C help boost immunity. They are naturally antibacterial and so can eliminate a range of bacteria, especially those that affect the digestive system, such as salmonella. They can also increase the nutrient uptake from your food as you digest. The vitamin K they provide is critical for bone integrity and mineral density, especially for those dealing with osteoporosis or arthritis.

Chives

CILANTRO/CORIANDER

The cilantro plant (*Coriandrum sativum*) provides the herb's stems and leaves, plus the seeds that are known as the spice coriander. Both are essential to Mexican, Indian, and Asian cooking. The saponins contained in the plant can sometimes smell soapy. Cilantro originated in southern Europe, northern Africa, and southwestern Asia. It is a medium-sized herb with feathery leaves and small white or pale pink

CULINARY HERBS

flowers. The Greeks and Romans used it medicinally, and early Britons combined it with cumin and vinegar to preserve meat. It has antiseptic properties for treating mouth ulcers and antioxidants for preventing eye diseases. The seeds exceed antibiotics for combating salmonella-based ailments. The plant also inhibits gram-positive and gram-negative bacteria and contains dietary fiber, calcium, selenium, magnesium, iron, and manganese.

DILL

Dill (*Anethum graveolans*) is a delicate culinary herb that has a long medicinal history. It originated in the eastern Mediterranean and is now a popular addition to soups and to fish and potato dishes. It grows well in temperate regions, producing tall, frilly stems. Healers used it for relief from insomnia, digestive complaints, diarrhea, dysentery, menstrual disorders, respiratory issues, and various types of cancer. Its calcium content means it aids bone health, and its antimicrobial properties boost immunity. It is an anti-inflammatory that has been employed since ancient times to ease arthritis and gout. The seeds can also be used to freshen breath.

Dill

FENNEL

Fennel (*Foeniculum vulgare*) is an aromatic flowering plant that originated in the Mediterranean. This licorice-flavored hardy perennial features sleek, sturdy stems, feathery leaves, and yellow flowers; it can reach eight feet in height. The plant's beneficial volatile oils are responsible for its digestive, carminative, antiflatulent, and antioxidant properties. It has been used to relieve colic, treat ulcers and anemia, promote milk flow in nursing mothers, and expel wind. It is effective in treating high blood pressure and high cholesterol. Its seeds provide dietary fiber, and its flavonoid antioxidants battle free radicals. It contains vitamins A, B complex, C, and D, as well as copper, iron, calcium, potassium, manganese, and magnesium.

Fennel

GARLIC

This cousin to the onion, known in Asia for 6,000 years, is both a valued culinary staple and a versatile agent for health. *Allium sativum*, also called the "stinking rose," grows as a bulb with two-foot stems and globular pinkish flowers. Early healers used it to treat infections, indigestion, low libido, and even plague and leprosy. Modern research indicates its usefulness for regulating blood pressure, lowering triglycerides and bad cholesterol, reducing oxidative stress to blood vessels, and preventing blood clots. High intake may lower the risk of many cancers; its antibacterial and antiviral properties allow garlic to fight bacterial and viral infections.

GINGER

Referred to as a "gifts of the gods" by some early cultures, ginger (*Zingiber officinale*) served culinary, medicinal, and spiritual needs. It is a reed-like perennial with pinkish buds that mature to exotic yellow flowers. Ginger originated in Southeast Asia and soon naturalized in China, India, and the Middle East; as far back as 3000 BC it was being used to ease indigestion. Early healers used it to treat cold, flu, toothache, joint pain, and as protection against the plague. Modern medicine hailed its stomach calming qualities and its antioxidant and anti-inflammatory effects. It can be purchased fresh, dried, crushed, and powdered. A piece of ginger worn in an amulet is said to protect the health of the wearer.

Ginger

HIBISCUS

An annual of the tropics, the hibiscus plant (*Hibiscus sabdariffa*) likely originated in Egypt before naturalizing in other warm climates. The culinary variety, called roselle, produces buff flowers with maroon centers; its dried blossoms are used in cooking or to produce teas, sweet syrups, and jams. Nutritionally, hibiscus is rich in vitamin C, thiamin, and iron. Medicinally, it offers laxative, diuretic, antibacterial, and antiscorbutic properties. It is loaded with antioxidants that support the liver, reduce fevers, stimulate the appetite, and relieve colds and flu. Its anti-inflammatory benefits may help reduce the effects of metabolic syndrome—high cholesterol, high triglycerides, and high blood sugar combined with extra weight.

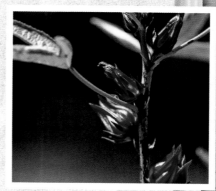

Hibiscus

HOPS

Hops are the female seed cones (strabiles) of the hop plant (*Humulus lupulus*), which are used to flavor and stabilize beer. This plant is a vigorous grower with climbing vines that can reach 20 feet or more. Originally cultivated in Germany in the 900s, hops have been used to ease anxiety, relieve stomach disorders, reduce menstrual cramps,

CULINARY HERBS

and induce sleep and relaxation. A flavonoid compound, xanthohumol, may have antiviral, anticlotting, anti-inflammatory, and antitumor activity. Hops extract is loaded with antioxidants that mimic the effects of a woman's own estrogen. Hops can increase production of digestive acids beneficial for bladder and urinary-tract infections.

LEMONGRASS

Now a staple of health-food stores, lemongrass (*Cymbopogon citratus*) has a long history as a flavoring in Asian cooking. This native of India and southern Asia is a tall perennial grass with fragrant, sword-like leaves that repel most insects but attract honeybees. Healers have used it to ease stomach pain, spasms, coughs, body aches, and fatigue. Studies show that lemongrass offers high levels of antioxidants and can aid digestion, lower high blood pressure, boost metabolism, burn fat, act as a tonic for skin and hair, and relieve menstrual pain. It is rich in vitamins B1, B5, and B6; in folic acid; and in the minerals potassium, zinc, calcium, iron, manganese, copper, and magnesium.

Lemongrass

LICORICE

This plant offers much more than a flavoring for candy. The licorice plant (*Glycyrrhiza glabra*), which is native to Europe and parts of Asia, is a tall, perennial legume that produces purple or lavender flowers. It is from the dried root that the actual herb is extracted. Licorice was once used by ancient cultures to treat coughs and colds—due to its anti-inflammatory, anti-allergic and expectorant qualities—and recent studies indicate it may be effective for treating gastric ulcers, chronic hepatitis, and Addison's disease (adrenal insufficiency). Other benefits include easing constipation and inflammation of the lungs, bowel, and skin, and bolstering immunity by raising levels of antiviral interferon.

Licorice sticks

MARJORAM

This piney-citrus kitchen favorite also has a long tradition as an herbal curative. Marjoram (*Origanum marjorana*), which likely originated in North Africa and Arabia, is a delicate

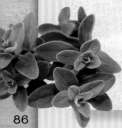

perennial with a downy stem, oval opposite leaves of grayish green, and tiny white or pink flowers. The herb is rich in vitamins A and C and is an important source of vitamin K. It was once used to treat stomach problems, staph infections, flu, typhoid, malaria, asthma, migraines, and body aches, and was believed to lower cholesterol and blood pressure, and stimulate circulation. Recent research validates many of these uses—the herb is brimming with antioxidants and phytonutrients and displays anti-inflammatory and antibacterial properties.

MINT

The genus *Mentha* features a number of medicinal herbs, including two with a long curative history: spearmint (*M. Spicata*) and peppermint (*M. piperita*). Typically mints have square stems and green serrated leaves, and produce delicate pinkish or lavender flowers. As culinary herbs, they mix well with other salad greens and make a pleasant, soothing tea. Mints act as appetite stimulants and palate cleansers, calm indigestion and heartburn, relieve the nausea of motion sickness, and ease the pain of headaches when applied to the forehead. Their pungent odor can clear up the congestion and coughing of colds or flu; for asthmatics, mint also acts as a relaxant.

Mint

OREGANO

Zesty, deeply aromatic oregano (*Origanum vulgare*) is prized by cooks and herbal healers alike. Native to Eurasia and the Mediterranean, this perennial features spade-shaped olive green leaves and spikes of small purple flowers. It is used to prepare sauces, vegetables, meat, fish, and pizza. Medicinally, it boosts immunity, and treats digestive issues, skin ailments, and fatigue. Its antibacterial qualities defend the body from digestive, urinary, and skin infections, its antioxidants relieve stress, and its fiber content eases digestion. It contains vitamins A, B6, C, E, and K, along with fiber, folate, iron, copper, magnesium, calcium, potassium, manganese, and the omega-3 fatty acids that balance cholesterol levels and reduce cardiovascular inflammation.

Oregano

ROSEMARY

Once valued by early healers, this popular culinary herb is used to flavor stuffing, grilled vegetables, and meat dishes. A woodsy perennial in the mint family, *Rosmarinus officinalis* originated in the coastal Mediterranean regions. Plants can reach five feet in height and display evergreen, needle-like leaves and pale flowers. Rosemary was once used to treat memory loss, sour stomach, diarrhea, and pain. Today, its antioxidant, anti-flammatory, and anticarcinogenic properties pose a threat to diseases that impact the immune

Rosemary

CULINARY HERBS

system; rosemary also combats bacterial infections such as *Helicobacter pylori*, which causes stomach ulcers and staph infections. Recent studies have found it stimulates brain activity in older adults, even those with advanced cognitive disorders such as Alzheimer's.

SAGE

This kitchen favorite, with its lemony scent, was employed by early healers as a digestive, gargle, nerve tonic, and poultice. *Salvia officinalis* is a perennial evergreen shrub in the mint family that originated in the Mediterranean. The plants reach two feet in height, with woolly leaves of gray-green and flowers of blue or cream. The ancient Egyptians, Greeks, Romans, and the healers of India valued it for increasing fertility, curing palsy, and as a brain tonic. It is known to have antibacterial, antifungal, antiviral, and astringent properties, and is used to treat diarrhea, colds, throat infections, hot flashes, and excess perspiration. It reduces outbreaks of oral or genital herpes and is showing effectiveness against Alzheimer's.

Sage

SORREL

Sorrel (*Rumex acetosa*) is a lemony-tasting garden herb that possesses immunity-boosting benefits. Originally a popular English herb, it eventually spread to the Continent. The plant reaches two feet in height, with fleshy stems, arrow-shaped leaves, and whorled spikes with reddish-green flowers. Sorrel's cooling properties were considered effective against "hot" ailments—inflammations, malaria fevers, and violent moods. It contains healthful flavonoids, antioxidants, and anthocyanins, and can be used to treat high blood pressure, heart disease, diabetes, and cancer. The herb's tannins clear nasal passages, and sorrel can also improve eyesight, boost immunity, strengthen bones, and slow aging. The herb is rich in vitamins C, A, and B9, and in potassium, magnesium, sodium, calcium, and iron.

TARRAGON

Sorrel

A favorite of French chefs and home cooks for its bittersweet anise-like flavor, tarragon (*Artemesia dracunculus*) originated in Siberia and western Asia. The shrub can reach four feet in height and displays lanceolate glossy leaves, narrow woody stems, and tiny yellowish blossoms. Natural healers valued this herb for stimulating appetite and easing indigestion, flatulence, and anorexia. It was also drunk as a tea to cure insomnia. Modern research has revealed the herb's true strength: tarragon is a powerhouse antioxidant, ridding the body of free radicals that damage RNA, DNA, and cell walls, and cause premature aging. It further supports heart health, can lower bad cholesterol, and reduces tooth pain. It is also rich in valuable phytonutrients.

TEA

Hot or cold, tea is a restorative beverage with a range of health benefits. Tea comes from an evergreen shrub (Camellia sinensis), harvested from either a narrow-leaf variety that grows in the cool mountains of central China and Japan, or from a broad-leaf variety that prefers the moist, tropical climate of northeast India and west-central China. Both varieties display glossy green leaves and small white flowers. The four main teas— black, green, oolong, and white—all offer health benefits, including high levels of antioxidants, sodium, proteins, and carbohydrates. Tea has been used to treat high cholesterol, breast cancer, diarrhea, asthma, cardiovascular issues, skin irritations, and cold sores.

Tea plant

THYME

Piquant thyme (*Thymus vulgaris*), a cousin of oregano, originated in the Mediterranean and parts of Africa. It is a small, bushy, woody shrub that displays small, aromatic gray-green leaves and pink or purple flowers in clusters. In the kitchen, thyme is found in both the bouquet garni and *herbes de Provence*. The Egyptians used it in the embalming process; the Greeks burned it as incense. Thyme's main active ingredient, thymol, acts as an antifungal and antiviral, bolstering the immune system. An impressive number of antioxidants stimulate production of red blood cells, support cardiovascular function, and lower blood pressure. Its expectorant and anti-inflammatory qualities make it ideal for treating colds and flu.

WATERCRESS

This peppery-tasting aquatic plant (*Nasturtium officinale*), which grows in meandering streams, is native to Europe and Asia and is related to mustard and radish. It has hollow stems that enable it to float, scalloped bright-green leaves, and clusters of small white flowers. Greeks and Romans used it to treat respiratory ailments and to make a healthful spring tonic. It is now used to regulate cholesterol and blood pressure, support the heart, increase bone strength, fight off infection, maintain connective tissue, and prevent iron deficiency. It reduces free radical damage to DNA and displays anticancer properties. Watercress is rich in vitamin K, vitamin A, vitamin C, riboflavin, vitamin B6, and calcium.

MEDICINAL HERBS

Even if it took humans many centuries to determine that certain plants they consumed helped cure disease and illness, once the link was established, these medicinal herbs soon became integrated into cultures across the globe, and remain so today.

ALFALFA

This flowering perennial in the pea family—the young plant resembles clover—originated in Asia, but is now grown worldwide as a forage crop. The Arabs, who fed it to their prized horses, named it *al-fac-facah* or "father of all foods." Traditional healers used it to treat the kidneys, bladder, and prostate, and to cleanse the bowels. The leaves offer antiarthritic, antidiabetic, and antiasthmatic properties. Studies suggest the plant may reduce cholesterol

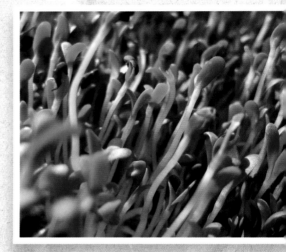

Alfalfa

levels and boost the immune system. Nutritionally, alfalfa contains chlorophyll; carotene; protein; a host of minerals, including calcium, iron, and magnesium; all the B vitamins; and vitamins C, D, E, and K.

ALOE

Aloe vera is a stemless succulent that grows wild in many tropical regions. The gel has long been used by numerous cultures as a treatment for burns and skin irritations. The leaves are thick, fleshy, and

Aloe

spear-like; in summer the plant produces pendulous yellow blossoms on tall spikes. Its medicinal properties include antioxidant, antimicrobial, and antibacterial. Research supports the plant's ability to soothe first- or second-degree burns and to treat genital herpes and psoriasis. Aloe juice is also an effective remedy for acid indigestion. The plant contains more than 75 active compounds, including vitamins, minerals, enzymes, sugars, amino acids, and fatty acids.

ANGELICA

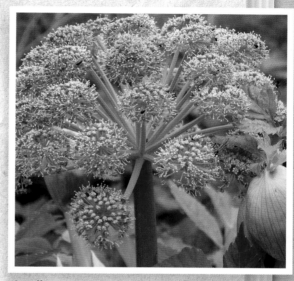

The genus *Angelica* features tall, robust, aromatic plants that likely originated in the temperate coastal regions of the Northern Hemisphere. The plants can reach to nine feet in height, with large bipinnate leaves and umbels made of greenish-white flowers. *Angelica archangelica* is probably native to Syria; the roots, leaves, and seeds are used to treat colds, urinary ailments, indigestion, and anxiety. In Chinese medicine, *Angelica sinensis* is known as

Angelica

dong quai, or female ginseng. It may help to reduce pain, dilate blood vessels, stimulate or relax uterine muscles, and enhance the immune system. The dried root is rich in vitamin B12, zinc, thiamine, riboflavin, potassium, magnesium, and iron.

ARNICA

This topical healing herb *(Arnica montana)* is a member of the large Compositae, or sunflower, family. Native to the mountains of Europe and Siberia, it is now also found in North America. It has fleecy, green leaves with daisy-like, yellow-orange blossoms. Since the fifteenth century, the flower heads have been used to make soothing creams, salves, and ointments for treating muscle aches, strains, sprains, and bruises— although it is never used on

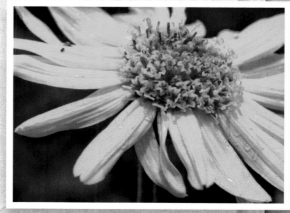

Arnica

MEDICINAL HERBS

or near any open wounds. The plant contains selenium and manganese, both valuable antioxidants.

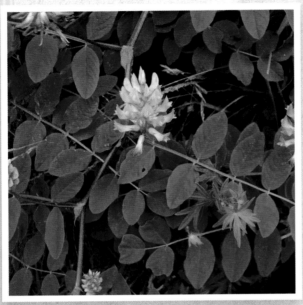

Astragalus

ASTRAGALUS

Astragalus (*Astragalus membranaceus*), also known as milkvetch, originated in Asia. It is part of the pea family, with green pinnate leaves and lipped flowers in pink and yellow. The firm, fibrous root's yellow core is the source of the healing herb. Known in China as *huang qi*, it has been used medicinally for more than 2,000 years. Western healers prescribe it to reverse the effects of aging on the immune system. As an antiviral and antibacterial agent, it is also able to ward off colds and flu, benefit the liver, lungs, and spleen, and encourage new tissue growth.

BURDOCK

Burdock (*Arctium lapa*) is a wildflower that originated in Europe and Asia and came to America with French and English settlers. This tall, stout plant features large, wedge-shaped leaves and purple flowers that mature into thistle-like fruits. These give off notoriously clingy burrs. The dried root of the plant has been used for centuries as a blood purifier, to treat skin infections such as boils, to clear up acne or psoriasis, and to promote circulation. A burdock-leaf poultice is excellent for treating gout. Burdock root contains a high concentration of inulin, which strengthens the liver, and mucilage, which soothes the GI tract. It also possesses antioxidant, antibacterial, and antifungal properties.

Burdock

CALENDULA

Calendula (*Calendula officinalis*), or pot marigold, is native to southwestern Asia, western Europe, Macronesia, and the Mediterranean. Saint Hildegard of Bingen was likely the first to cultivate the herb, which became a mainstay of European herbal studies. With its anti-inflammatory, antimicrobial, and antiviral properties, it is considered one of the best remedies for slow-healing wounds or ulcers. It is also prescribed for abdominal cramps, constipation, women's reproductive issues, sore throats, diaper rash, chapped lips, or split skin. In ayurvedic medicine the herb is used on minor wounds, eye irritations, and bee stings. Called *jin zhan ju* in Chinese medicine, calendula is used to support healthy skin.

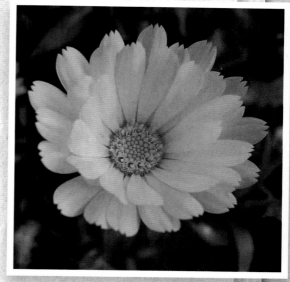

Calendula

CHAMOMILE

Matricaria chamomilla, or German chamomile, is the variety typically used by herbalists. This daisy-like plant is native to Europe, Asia, and North Africa; it reaches three feet in height, with green, feathery leaves and florets of small white flowers. Chamomile tea is known for its stomach-calming and sleep-inducing qualities, but the herb has also been used to treat colds, hay fever, inflammation, muscle spasms, migraines, menstrual disorders, gastrointestinal issues, skin irritations, and hemorrhoids. It possesses

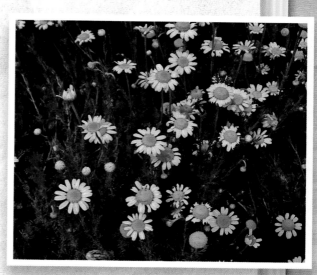

Chamomile

antiseptic, anti-inflammatory, and emollient qualities. It can be taken in the form of teas, tinctures, lotions, capsules, or drops. *Chamaemelum nobile*, known as Roman or English chamomile, also has medicinal uses.

MEDICINAL HERBS

CLARY SAGE

Clary sage (*Salvia sclarea*) is a cousin of garden sage. This perennial or biennial herb originated in the Mediterranean region and central Asia. It grows to three feet in height, with sturdy, hairy stems and clumping purple flowers. In the Middle Ages, its mucilaginous properties led to its use as an eyewash and aid to clear sight. It has both anti-inflammatory and antioxidant properties, making it a powerful cholesterol fighter. It also helps to treat stress and poor circulation. Among the herb's chief chemical components are sclareol, which has shown potential for fighting leukemia, and linalyl acetate, which reduces skin irritations and rashes.

COMFREY

Russian comfrey *(Symphytum x uplandicum)* has a long history as a curative and a garden booster. Native to the riverbanks of Europe, the plant is now found in North America and western Asia. It bears broad, hairy leaves and small bell-like flowers in cream or purple; the turnip-like root is black. Comfrey, once known as boneset, was used to treat broken bones, sprains, strains, and arthritis as well as for bronchial problems, gastric distress, and varicose ulcers. The herb contains allantoin, believed to stimulate skin-cell growth and reduce inflammation. Comfrey should only be used topically as a salve or poultice, or as an essential oil.

DANDELION

Few weeds offer the nutritional and healing attributes of the dandelion (*Taraxacum officinale*), which originated in Eurasia. The plant can reach 15 inches in height, with oblong, jagged leaves and tiny yellow florets. The leaves are valuable detoxifiers, high in beta-carotene, fiber, vitamin C, potassium, calcium, and iron. The plant was effective for treating infections and liver problems, as a diuretic

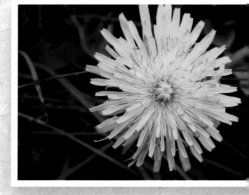

Dandelion

and laxative, and to improve digestion. Modern research confirms the presence of a number of flavonoids with antioxidant, anti-inflammatory, antitumor, and immunity-boosting properties. Dandelions have the potential to reduce the risk of cancer, control diabetes, aid in weight loss, treat gallbladder disorders, lower blood pressure, and treat urinary infections.

Some common names include lion's tooth, cankerwort, milk witch, yellow gowan, Irish daisy, monkshead, priest's crown, puffball, faceclock, pee-a-bed, wet-a-bed, swine's snout, white endive, and wild endive.

ECHINACEA

A longtime herbal remedy, *Echinacea purpurea* is native to North America. It can reach four feet in height, displaying coarse, often hairy leaves and cone-shaped heads with purple rays, or petals. Herbalists consider it a natural curative and wellness booster and utilize all of the plant—flowers, leaves, and roots. Most of its chemical constituents— essential oils, inulin, flavonoids, and vitamin C— augment immunity. The herb is also used for treating colds, flu, sinusitis, strep throat, whooping cough, bowel pain, and headaches. Research indicates that the herb's phytochemicals could be valuable for combating brain cancer tumors. Echinacea makes a safe,

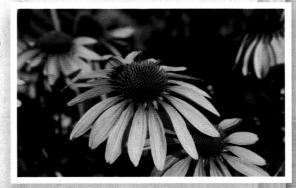

Echinacea

mild, natural laxative and its anti-inflammatory properties are useful against rheumatoid arthritis and uveitis.

The flower's spiky brownish central disk is responsible for its common name: *echinacea* derives from the Greek *ekhinos*, or "hedgehog," because it resembles a spiny animal.

ELDER

Sambucus nigra is native to Europe and North America. It is a large shrub with pinnate, serrated leaves and creamy, fragrant blossoms that mature into deep-purple berries. Elder was often referred to as the "medicine chest of the country people"—healers used the flowers and berries (other parts of the plant are toxic) to make healthful cordials and to treat respiratory, urinary, and digestive-tract ailments. Modern research revealed elder's antiseptic, antibacterial, antiviral, and anti-inflammatory properties. The plant's antioxidant bioflavonoids can ease allergies and regulate blood-glucose levels. Its triterpenoids offer analgesic, anti-inflammatory, and anticancer benefits. Elder is also

MEDICINAL HERBS

effective against hospital pathogens like staphylococcus. Elderberries need to be cooked prior to use.

The name *elder* comes from the Anglo-Saxon *aeld*, or "fire." In primitive dwellings, the hollowed stems were used to build up fires.

EVENING PRIMROSE

This herb, with its long history as a curative, is also welcomed in the garden. The plant (*Oenothera biennis*) produces an upright stem with narrow lanceloate leaves and buttery-yellow flowers. Traditional healers employed it to regulate hormones and nourish hair and nails; Native Americans used almost the

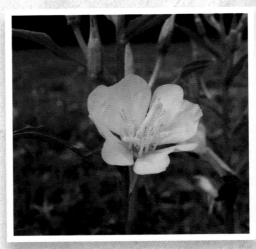

Evening primrose

whole plant as food and medicine. Today, research has revealed that evening primrose oil contains unusually high concentrations of GLA (gamma-linolenic acid), which gives the plant the potential to address hyperactivity in children and aging problems in adults; treat rheumatoid arthritis, eczema, and heart disease; and ease symptoms of menopause, Multiple sclerosis, obesity, PMS, and schizophrenia.

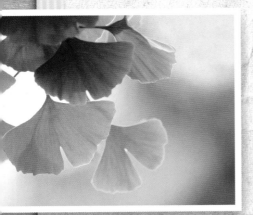

Ginkgo

GINKGO

Often called living fossils, ginkgo trees (*Ginkgo biloba*) originated in China, where they appear in fossil remains that go back 270 million years. The trees grow from 60 to 100 feet and have lobed, fan-shaped leaves. Females produce slender flowers and pink and orange seeds, while males later display small pollen-bearing cones. Used as a tonic in Chinese medicine for millennia, the leaf extract's many health claims are now in dispute. Still, in studies the herb helped reduce the uncontrolled movements (tardive dyskinesia) caused by antipsychotic drugs, eased migraine pain, and improved concentration in children with ADHD. Ginkgo also stabilized or slowed the mental deterioration associated with Alzheimer's, dementia, and cognitive impairment.

Ginkgo is also known as the maidenhair tree, the fossil tree, kew tree, or silver apricot—which translate into *gin kyo* in Japanese,

GINSENG

Chinese ginseng *(Panax ginseng)*, with its long reign as a leading remedy, continues to gain new advocates. The slow-growing perennial originated in the Manchurian mountains and is now found in cooler temperate zones. This small plant displays serrated leaflets and small

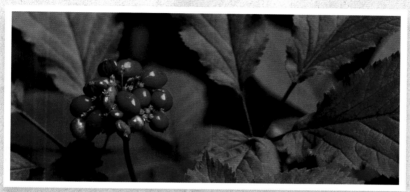

Ginseng

greenish flowers that form red berries. The pale, fleshy root contains ginsenosides and gintonins that benefit the cardiovascular, central nervous, and immune systems. American ginseng (*P. quinquefolius*) was once used to treat headaches, fevers, coughs, and wounds. Some may question the herb's touted benefits, but clinical evidence indicates it is effective for treating high blood pressure, diabetes, hyperlipidemia, heart failure, fatigue, and memory loss.

The plant's genus name, *Panax*, is Greek for "all-healing," a measure of how much early civilizations revered this herb.

GOJI BERRY

Hailed as one of nature's "superfoods," nutrient-rich goji berries come from two species of boxthorn, *Lycium barbarum* or *L. chinense*.

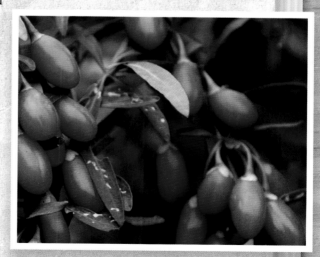

Goji berry

Also called wolfberry, the sweetly tart fruits originated in Asia. These perennials range in height from three to nine feet, with small lanceolate

MEDICINAL HERBS

or ovate leaves and pink or purple trumpet-shaped flowers. Healers value the fruit's ability to increase vigor, fight disease, and improve mood. Modern research cites their benefits to the GI and urinary tracts, and the cardiovascular, respiratory, and musculoskeletal systems. They boosts skin and eye health and may be able to increase the potency of flu vaccines in seniors, improve sexual ability, and cause tumors to undergo "cell suicide."

GOLDENSEAL

Goldenseal *(Hydrastis canadensis)* is native to North America. This low-growing woodland plant produces a pair of hairy, lobed, palmate leaves and a single greenish flower that forms a berry. Indigenous tribes used the dried root to treat colds and digestive issues, and European settlers also employed it for fatigue, fever, bleeding, and urinary problems. Goldenseal has retained much of its healing reputation into modern times, where it is acknowledged for its antibacterial and antifungal properties. It also contains vitamins A, C, E, and B complex, calcium, iron, and manganese.

HEARTSEASE

Known to gardeners as Johnny-jump-up, this flowering plant *(Viola tricolor)* is native to Europe. A small, creeping annual with petals of purple, yellow, and white, it is the progenitor of cultivated pansies. Medicinally, these plants have been used for thousands of years to relieve headaches and dizziness and to treat epilepsy, ulcers, and skin diseases. Today, heartsease is employed for its

THINK ABOUT IT!

In the emotionally rigid world of Victorian England, flowers were often used as secret symbols for different emotions. When you consider its folk names—heart's delight, tickle-my-fancy, Jack jump-up-and-kiss-me, come-and-cuddle me, and love-in-idleness—it's not surprising *Viola tricolor* represented loving remembrance and secret courtship.

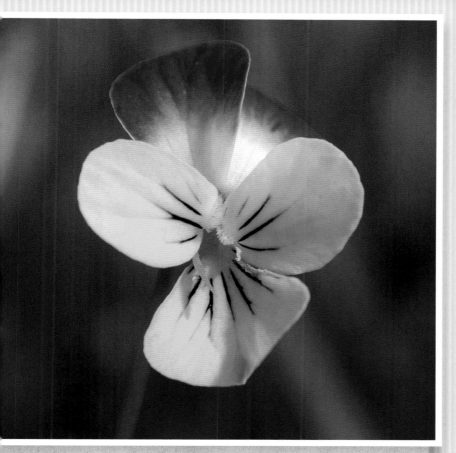

Heartsease

antimicrobial, antioxidant, and expectorant properties; it can help lower cholesterol and reduce risk of heart disease. It is also used to stabilize certain drugs.

LEMON BALM

Citrusy, aromatic lemon balm has a long history for easing stress and boosting brain power. This perennial mint (*Melissa officinalis*) originated in southern Europe and spread to central Asia. It may reach four feet in height, with heart-shaped, serrated leaves and delicate white flowers. Early healers used lemon balm—internally and as a tea—to increase appetite, ease pain, and support liver and digestive health. Today, lemon balm is well-regarded for its high levels of antioxidants and its eugenol, with antiseptic and anesthetic properties. Extracts of the herb had a measurable effect on lab-

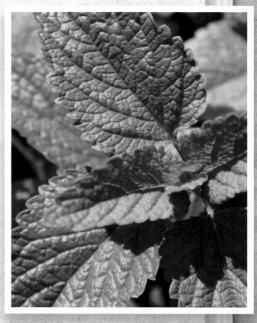

Lemon balm

MEDICINAL HERBS

caused stress in human subjects. As a facial balm, it boosts the body's defense against organisms that damage the complexion.

These richly aromatic plants are magnets for winged pollinators, and lemon balm's generic name, melissa, comes from the Greek for "honey bee."

MILK THISTLE

Milk thistle (*Silybum marianum*), which is native to the Mediterranean, can reach ten feet in height. The pale, hairy, green leaves sprout sharp spines along the margins; the flowers form spiky red or purple crowns. For millennia this herb was used to treat canker sores, headaches, vertigo, baldness, and disorders of the liver and gallbladder. It is now recognized for its ability to draw toxins from the body and decrease or reverse liver damage caused by medications, pollution, and exposure to heavy metals. It has potential for treating kidney and gallstones and the effects of chemotherapy.

The plant is rich in antioxidants and anti-inflammatories and vitamins C and E.

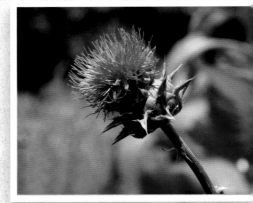

The name comes from the milky-white fluid that oozes from its crushed leaves—or possibly from the milky patches on the leaves.

Drinking a smoothie containing milk thistle before a night on the town, and again the next morning, is an effective way to prevent a hangover.

Milk thistle

MULLEIN

Mullein (*Verbascum thapsus*) is a tall-stalked garden favorite and a valued medicinal herb. Originally native to Europe and Asia, European settlers carried it to the New World, where Native Americans used it for skin and respiratory conditions. It ranges from three to nine feet in height; second-year plants send up a spike with small, pale flowers in yellow, orange, purple, blue, brown,

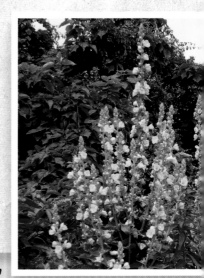

Mullein

and white. The plant was employed by ancient cultures to treat hemorrhoids, arthritis, ringworm, burns, tuberculosis, colds, pneumonia, allergies, and sore throats. Recent Irish research supports many of these uses—the leaf extract contains antiviral, antitumor, antifungal, and antibacterial qualities. The herb is also an anti-inflammatory and antispasmodic.

Mullein has many fanciful names: clown's lungwort, Bullock's lungwort, Our Lady's flannel, Adam's flannel, beggar's blanket, blanket herb, wild ice leaf, Aaron's rod, Jupiter's staff, Peter's staff, Jacob's staff, shepherd's staff, Cuddy's lungs, feltwort, fluffweed, hare's beart, and old man's beard.

PSYLLIUM

Psyllium (*Plantago psyllium*), or ispaghula, refers to several plants in the plantain family with mucilage-producing seeds. Native to northern India and Iran, it is a small annual with long narrow leaves and a tall stalk that produces tiny white flowers. These mature into small, dark, glossy seeds. In early Asian medicine, as now, psyllium was employed as a bulk-forming laxative—the husks

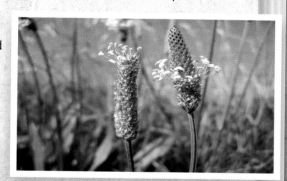

Psyllium

and seeds are considered soluble fiber, passing through the digestive tract without completely breaking down. Their mucilage content absorbs water, helping to soften stool, which makes the seeds effective for treating irritable bowel syndrome and hemorrhoids. Recent studies indicate psyllium may also lower triglycerides and blood glucose, control cholesterol, and aid in weight loss.

ROSE HIPS

Rose hips, the nutrient-laden fruits of the rose plant, have been part of folk medicine for hundreds of years, and were likely ingested by Stone Age humans. Roses are a perennial, woody flowering plant, mainly native to Asia. The bloom produces a rounded hip that ripens during late summer or fall. Not all

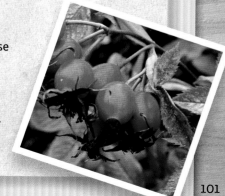

MEDICINAL HERBS

species produce large hips, but varieties that do include dog roses (*Rosa canina*), and common roses (*R. majalis*), both major sources of vitamin C. These impressive amounts of the vitamin give the immune system a boost and stimulate white blood cells. They also may reduce cholesterol and blood glucose levels, and eliminate free radicals.

Rose hips can be used to make herbal supplements, herbal teas, jellies, jams, marmalades, beverages, syrup, pie fillings, and wine.

SAINT-JOHN'S-WORT

Longtime herbal calmative, Saint-John's-wort (*Hypericum perforatum*) is a flowering plant native to the temperate regions of Europe and Asia. It can reach two feet in height and bears erect, woody-based stems and yellow, five-petaled flowers. Early cultures used the herb in tonics and to treat sores, inflammations, burns, sprains, and nerve pain. Practitioners of American eclectic medicine in the 1800s used it as a treatment for anxiety, nervous complaints, and depression, one of its chief uses today. When studies validated its effect on mild-to-moderate depression, it was then employed to treat anxiety, insomnia, seasonal affective disorder (SAD), hypothyroidism, shingles, menopausal symptoms, PMS, and bladder issues.

This plant has a long association with Saint John the Baptist—it traditionally flowers on Saint John's Day, June 24.

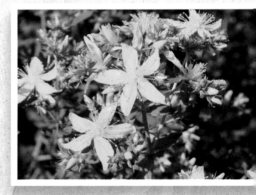

Saint-John's-wort

TEA TREE OIL

The tea tree (*Melaleuca alternifolia*), which is native to Australia, reaches an average height of 20 feet and features a bushy crown; papery whitish bark; long, smooth, oil-rich leaves; and soft masses of cream-colored or white flowers on spikes. For a hundred years, Australians have used the oil to treat fungal nail infections, acne, and psoriasis. The indigenous

Tea tree

Bundjalung people of eastern Australia inhaled the oil's vapors to treat coughs and colds and applied the crushed leaves to wounds. Today, this essential oil—with its antiseptic, antibacterial, antifungal, antiviral, and antimicrobial properties—treats acne outbreaks, athlete's foot, and jock itch; combats foot odor; and relieves chicken pox rash and cold sores.

The fluffy blossoms account for the folk name snow-in-summer. Other names include narrow-leaved paperbark, narrow-leaved tea-tree, and narrow-leaved ti-tree.

VALERIAN

Valerian (*Valeriana officinalis*) is native to Europe and Asia and became an introduced species in North America. It can reach five feet in height and bears deeply toothed green leaves and sweetly scented pink or white flowers. It has a long medicinal history—the Greeks and Romans used it for insomnia, indigestion, anxiety, urinary infections, and liver complaints, and Indian, Arab, and Chinese physicians wrote of its curative powers. Today, healers make preparations from the roots, rhizomes, and stolons to induce sleep and to treat migraines, high blood pressure, anxiety, and muscle cramps. The herb has antiseptic, anticonvulsant, and analgesic qualities, and contains the compound

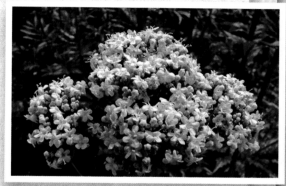

Valerian

gamma-aminobutyric acid (GABA), a receptor that may boost brain power and lower stress.

WILLOW BARK

A potent analgesic called salicin, perhaps the oldest known to humans, is derived from the bark of the willow tree. Willows range in size from tall tress to spreading shrubs, and are native to Europe, Asia, and North America. The species most often harvested is the white willow (*Salix alba*), followed by the purple willow (*S. purpurea*). These trees produce thin, lance-shaped leaves, and bristling, tubular flowers called catkins. Ancient cultures chewed the bark to ease painful injuries, childbirth, and headaches, and to lower fever. It possesses anti-inflammatory, antiseptic, and immunity-boosting properties and is now used to treat migraines, back spasms, menstrual cramps, and irritable bowel syndrome, and to reduce the swelling of tendonitis.

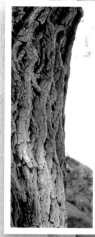

Willow bark

AROMATIC HERBS

These deeply scented herbs have for millennia been the sources of perfume, incense, cleansers, disinfectants, and many essential oils. When it comes to treating health concerns, they are used topically or via inhalation, rarely through ingestion.

BEE BALM

This lanky garden favorite (*Monarda spp.*) is a midsummer bloomer that also has time-tested medicinal uses. The perennial mint is native to

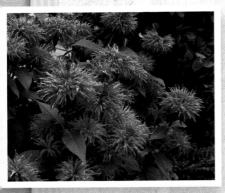

the eastern United States—it was a valued treatment for infections in Native American culture—but has spread to parts of Europe and Asia. The plant can reach two or more feet in height; has a grooved, square stem; paired, toothed leaves; and clustered tubular flowers in rich colors. Healers use the leaves and flowers to ease gas and as a diuretic, stimulant, and antiseptic. It can be taken as an infusion to relieve colds, headaches, gastric and menstrual pain, and insomnia, and when inhaled as steam, it quickly loosens the congestion of bronchitis.

Bee balm

BERGAMOT ORANGE

With its woodsy citrus odor, the essential oil of bergamot orange is used in one-third to one-half of commercial perfumes. It is distilled from the rind of the orange, the fruit of a small winter-blooming tree (*Citrus bergamia*) found in Southeast Asia. For many years it has been used to improve circulation, stimulate hormone secretion, maintain metabolism, elevate mood, aid digestion, prevent infection, and ease pain. It also helps to heal skin irritations and eliminate scarring. The extract psoralen was once used in sunblocks, but was found to be carcinogenic in light. Today it is combined with UVA light as PUVA therapy for healing skin ailments such as psoriasis and eczema.

Bergamot orange

EUCALYPTUS

More than 700 species of eucalyptus, or gum trees, occur throughout Australia. The genus originated in South America, where it is no longer native. They are mostly evergreens featuring lanceolate, petiolate, and alternate leaves with a waxy or glossy green surface. The flowers have multiple fluffy stamens in white, yellow, pink, or red and cone-shaped fruits that release rod-shaped seeds. The bark is heavily textured. The oil offers anti-inflammatory, antimicrobial, and antibacterial properties and is used to treat wounds, muscle aches, joint pain, mental exhaustion, and skin problems. One organic compound, cineole—the object of more than a thousand studies—can reduce inflammation and pain and even destroy leukemia cells.

HYSSOP

Minty, slightly bitter hyssop (*Hyssopus officinalis*) may be used to

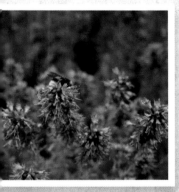

Hyssop

flavor foods but it is also valued in the production of cologne and administered as a warm tea against colds and flu. The plant, which is native to southern Europe and the Middle East, is a semi-woody evergreen mint that can reach three feet in height, with square stems, oblong leaves, and whorls of scented bluish-purple flowers. Used for purification in biblical times, the herb today is known to have antiseptic, antispasmodic, antidepressant, expectorant, and diuretic properties. It improves circulation and treats female complaints, and its astringent qualities lend it to healing skin conditions such as dermatitis and eczema.

JASMINE

Long a symbol of seduction and sensuality, richly scented jasmine (*Jasmimum spp.*) is a garden favorite. Native to Persia and India, this evergreen shrub is a climber that can attain 40 feet in length. It bears pinnate green leaves and cascading clusters of white star-shaped flowers. Early Asian physicians esteemed jasmine's leaves and flowers for treating headache, insomnia, joint problems, gallstones, skin outbreaks, and scabies. The herb is recognized today as astringent, antibacterial, and antiviral; its oil is beneficial to aging skin and will heal sores and abscesses when combined with sesame oil. Studies in Tokyo indicate the herb can increase alertness and stimulate brain waves.

AROMATIC HERBS

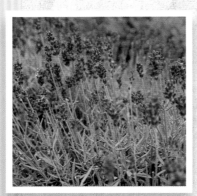

Lavender

LAVENDER

Lavender's role ranges from a garden staple and culinary flavoring to a medicinal oil and insect repellent. The two most popular species are English lavender (*Lavendula angustifolia*) and French lavender (*L. stoechas* or *L. dentata*). Native to the Mediterranean, this hardy evergreen shrub bears narrow gray-green leaves and pinkish purple flowers on spikes. The Egyptians applied it as perfume and included it in the mummification process. Healers have used it, topically or inhaled, against insomnia, anxiety, depression, digestive problems, headaches, toothaches, and sprains, and for healing burns. Diffused lavender oil may prevent cellular damage that can lead to cancer and protect the body from the components of diabetes.

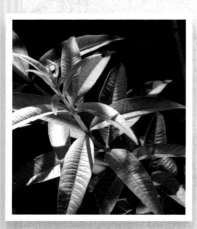

Lemon verbena

LEMON VERBENA

Often known as the "queen of the lemon-scented herbs," lemon verbena (*Aloysia citrodora*) is native to western South America. When the Spanish introduced it to Europe, it became a vital raw material for the perfume trade. The plant is a deciduous shrub that can reach six feet in height and produces glossy, lanceolate leaves and clustering, aromatic, small white or purple flowers on panicles. Once used as a sedative and to relieve stomach and joint pain, asthma, colds and hemorrhoids, it is known to possess anti-inflammatory, antispasmodic, and antioxidant qualities. Today, it is used to aid digestion, relieve arthritis pain, reduce tension, and as an expectorant.

PATCHOULI

This herb's distinctive acrid scent is reminiscent of the 1960s counterculture, but it also has a respected curative history. Originally found in Southeast Asia, it now grows in many parts of the tropics. *Pogostemon cablin* is an evergreen perennial shrub in the mint family that features serrated leaves and small pinkish-white flowers. For millennia, healers have used this herb to treat skin ailments, heal wounds, and reduce scarring. It provides mood-enhancing effects and possesses antidepressant, antiseptic, astringent, and aphrodisiac properties. In lab tests in India, the plant displayed its antibacterial and antifungal qualities by destroying 20 out of 22 bacterial strains and all 12 fungal strains it was exposed to.

RUE

Also known as herb-of-grace, rue (*Ruta graveolens*) is an ornamental and medicinal herb with a pungent, soothing scent. Originally native to the Balkan Peninsula, it is now found around the world. The plant reaches three feet in height and bears velvety bluish leaves and bright-yellow flowers that mature into fruit. Rue was once thought to heighten creativity and improve eyesight, making it a favorite of artists like Leonardo da Vinci and Michelangelo. Modern healers recommend it for treating headaches, joint pain, insomnia, nerves, stomach cramps, and renal problems as well as skin ailments such as psoriasis. There is some indication that rue, when combined with certain other herbs, may possess antiviral qualities.

SPIKENARD

Sweetly anise-scented spikenard (*Nardostachys jatamansi*) originated in the Himalayas and was valued in ayurvedic and Greco-Arab medicine as an additive to perfumes and incense, as an essential oil, and for treating insomnia, birthing problems, and headaches. The plant grows to three feet in height and displays green lanceolate leaves and dense clusters of pink, bell-shaped blooms. The root is dried and steam distilled to create the aromatic oil. Healers advise using spikenard oil as a rub for easing nausea, as an inhaled sedative to calm stress, and as an antibacterial facial massage to banish wrinkles. A drop of the oil after a meal will banish indigestion and act as a laxative.

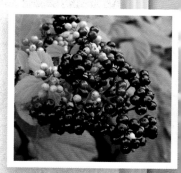

Spikenard

THINK ABOUT IT!
When sweet woodruff dries, its odor of honey and new-mown hay intensifies, making it an ideal addition to potpourris and sachets.

SWEET WOODRUFF

This shade-loving perennial, which is native to North Africa, Europe and western Asia, has been used as a culinary, aromatic, and healing herb. Sweet woodruff (*Galium odoratum*) forms low, dense mats; the plants display whorls of deep-green leaves and tiny white star-shaped flowers. Early physicians used it to treat liver problems and as a calmative. Today, natural healers recommend it for preventing lung, liver, stomach, and gallbladder disorders, to relieve insomnia and headaches, and as a diuretic. Direct topical applications of the anti-inflammatory leaves are said to help treat skin diseases, swelling, wounds, vein problems, and hemorrhoids.

HEALING SPICES

Many spices are a match for herbs when it comes to treating disease, healing wounds, soothing irritation, and easing pain. A number of medicinal spices can be obtained as essential oils, others can be found in supplement form.

ANISEED

This flowering plant, *Pimpinella anisum*, has been cultivated in the Mediterranean and western Asia for thousands of years. Reaching two feet in height, the herb's leaves are lobed at the base and feathery on the stem. The tiny white flowers form umbels and mature into small gray-brown fruit. The spice possesses a licorice flavor that is aromatic and fruity, the result of the compound anethole. Aniseed was highly regarded for its healing qualities—the Egyptians took it as a diuretic, the Greeks for pain. Today it is used to improve digestion, relieve asthma symptoms, reduce phlegm and inflammation, soothe skin irritations, increase metabolism, and improve heart health.

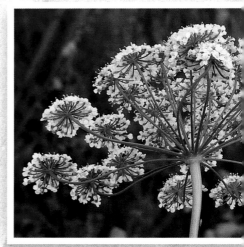

Aniseed

BLACK PEPPER

This "king of spices" was once used as a form of money and was presented to the gods during religious rituals. Black pepper (*Piper nigrum*) originated in Kerala, India, and is a woody vine that produces clusters of small white flowers, which form small red berries known as peppercorns. The spice was once applied medicinally against scourges such as scarlet fever, smallpox, and cholera, but today it is used to stimulate circulation, ease respiratory ailments, treat joint or muscle pain, increase metabolism, and improve immunity. The piperine in the plant acts as a painkiller, while its antioxidants combat free radicals, and the alkaloid capsaicin increases sweating and urination, speedily removing toxins from the body.

CARDAMOM

This densely aromatic spice, the third most expensive after saffron and vanilla, is made of seeds from plants native to India, Bhutan, Indonesia, and Nepal. True or green cardamom (*Elettaria cardamomum*) has a sweet flavor. Black cardamom (*Amomum subulatum*) has a dark, smoky flavor. Part of both ayurvedic and Chinese traditional medicine, it's been used as a remedy for tooth and gum infections, throat ailments, inflamed eyelids, and gallstones. It is known to protect the gastrointestinal tract, control cholesterol levels, and treat urinary and respiratory infections. It can help control muscle spasms, inhibit the growth of microbes, and may have cancer-fighting potential. This spice is also rich in vitamins and minerals.

CAYENNE

This fiery gift to Europe from Central America has a long list of health benefits. Cayenne peppers can be red, green, or yellow and are the fruit of the chili plant (*Capsicum annuum*), a small perennial shrub with off-white or purplish flowers. First grown around 5000 BC, they are among the oldest cultivated plants. Indigenous people used cayenne to treat heartburn, fever, sore throat, paralysis, hemorrhoids, and nausea. The capsaicin in cayenne eases aches by depleting the pain-causing neurotransmitters in nerve endings. In studies, capsaicin also reduced heart arrhythmias, stimulated blood flow, and inhibited the growth of prostate cancer cells, and its beneficial compound, CAY-1, suppressed more than 16 fungal strains.

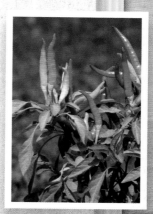
Cayenne peppers

Alternate names include cow-horn pepper, red hot chili pepper, aleva, bird pepper, and Guinea pepper. The common name is taken from Cayenne, the capital city of French Guiana.

CELERY SEED

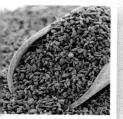
Celery seeds

Once valued by ayurvedic and Asian physicians, celery seed (*Apium graveolens*) was also part of early Mediterranean and medieval European folk medicine. The vegetable is native to southern Europe, displaying sturdy fleshy stems, wide segmented leaves, and airy umbels of white flowers. The aromatic oval seeds are used in the cuisines of Germany, Italy, and Russia. The herb has been used to improve cardiovascular health, lower blood pressure, and treat arthritis and liver ailments, colds, flu, toothache, backache, and indigestion.

AROMATIC HERBS

The seeds possess carminative, antibacterial, antiseptic, sedative, aphrodisiac, stimulant, and diuretic qualities, and are rich in antioxidants and in the beneficial, vanilla-scented compound coumarin, which is the source of their scent and taste.

CINNAMON

This warm, sweet kitchen favorite is harvested from the bark of two evergreen trees: Ceylon cinnamon, or true cinnamon (*Cinnamomum verum*), and cassia, or Chinese cinnamon (*C. aromaticum*). Early medicinal use dates back to at least 2000 BC. The spice is rich in antioxidants and effective for treating muscle spasms, vomiting, diarrhea,

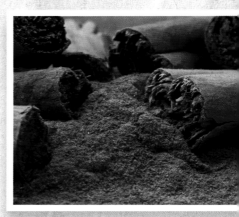

Cinnamon

colds, infections, loss of appetite, and erectile dysfunction. Research indicates the spice may also lower blood pressure, reduce cholesterol and triglycerides, improve glucose and lipid levels, treat bacterial and fungal infections, slow the development of Alzheimer's disease, combat HIV-1 and HIV-2, and help stop the destructive onslaught of multiple sclerosis.

CLOVES

Now synonymous with the winter holidays, cloves (*Syzygium aromaticum*) have been a valued remedy for thousands of years. The clove itself is the unopened flower bud of the clove tree, a smooth-barked evergreen that reaches 50 feet in height. These natives of the Indonesian Maluku Islands were introduced to Europe in the fourth century and used to cover the taste of spoiled meat. Cloves display potent antioxidant, anti-inflammatory, and antimicrobial properties and are excellent for treating stomach ailments, maintaining bone density, lowering risk of GI tract cancers, easing joint and tooth pain, boosting the immune system, and possibly controlling blood sugar levels. They are rich in both vitamins and minerals.

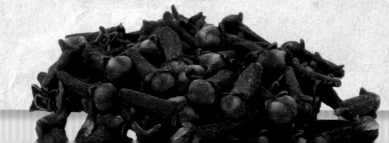

CUMIN

Worldwide, earthy, nutty cumin (*Cuminum cyminum*) is the second most popular spice after black pepper. The oval, yellowish seeds come from a small, slender-stemmed plant that produces white and pink clusters of flowers. Cumin originated in the Mediterranean and was used by the Egyptians for embalming. It is a potent antioxidant that can heal acne, rashes, and boils; its vitamin E content preserves the complexion by combating wrinkles, age spots, and sagging skin. It also has antimicrobial and antifungal properties, acts as a natural laxative, breaks up respiratory congestion, and speeds up secretion of detoxifying enzymes. It contains vitamins B1, B2, B3, C, and E and is high in fiber and iron.

JUNIPER BERRY

Juniper berries are the female seed cones of various junipers, most commonly *Juniperus communis*, an evergreen that originated in Asia, Canada, and northern Europe. It can be a dense shrub or a tree that reaches 40 feet in height. These tart, piney berries, which are popular additions to European game dishes and a flavoring for gin, also provide medicinal benefits—their antimicrobial and antifungal properties can destroy widespread gram-positive and gram-negative bacteria; as a

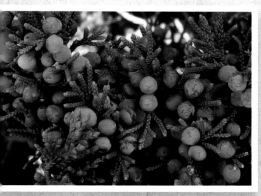

diuretic they can relieve bloating, reduce water retention, lower blood pressure, and remove extra salts; and they also flush out urinary bacteria and toxins. They contain high levels of antioxidants that can help combat cancer, heart disease, and arthritis.

Juniper berries

MACE/NUTMEG

Earthy, sweet nutmeg is the kernel of the nutmeg tree (*Myristica fragrans*), while a powdered seasoning called mace comes from the waxy red covering of the seed, or aril. This tall evergreen is native to the Maluku Islands in Indonesia, also home to cloves. The tree produces large, glossy, oval leaves and apricot-like drupes. Nutmeg has been valued by healers for millennia, as a brain tonic and for treating depression and anxiety, abdominal pain and inflammation, sleeplessness, and nausea, and for cleansing toxins from the liver and kidneys. It contains the compounds myristicin and macelignan, which are known to shield the brain from degenerative diseases such as Alzheimer's. Nutritionally, nutmeg contains potassium, calcium, iron, and manganese.

AROMATIC HERBS

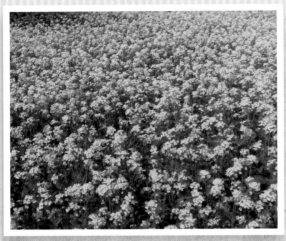

Mustard

MUSTARD

Mustard (*Brassica sp.*, *Sinapis sp.*) possibly dates back to Stone Age China. Mild white mustard was native to the Mediterranean region, spicy brown oriental mustard came from the Himalayan foothills, and intense black mustard originated in southern Europe and south Asia. All three have been called "superfoods" by nutritionists. They are a rich source of vitamin A, folate, calcium, magnesium, phosphorus, and potassium. Mustard has been used to treat asthma and rheumatoid arthritis, clear congestion, lower high blood pressure, limit migraines, and even inhibit the growth of stomach, colon, and cervical cancers. The seeds stimulate production of enzymes that protect the skin against psoriasis and help to heal the lesions.

SAFFRON

This delicate spice is made from the red-orange stigmas and styles of the saffron crocus (*Crocus sativus*), which are harvested by hand. This labor-intensive process makes saffron the most expensive spice by weight. Native to southwestern Asia, the plant ranges from 8 to 12 inches in height and bears narrow green leaves with white stripes and up to four purple flowers. Based on a Greek fresco, medicinal saffron goes back at least 3,500 years. Healers use it to suppress appetites, ease mild depression, reduce stress, soothe upset stomachs, and as an aphrodisiac for women with low libido. Its anti-inflammatory properties help reduce the pain of sports injuries and arthritis.

This versatile spice contains more than 150 volatile compounds and many micronutrients.

STAR ANISE

Sweet-scented star anise (*Illicium verum*) is native to southern China and northeast Vietnam; it grows on a medium-sized evergreen tree that bears large, glossy green leaves and decorative white flowers. The dark-brown pods have eight carpels (dried fruits) radiating out like a star. Early physicians used it as a stimulant and to treat coughs and colic, ease rheumatism and menstrual cramps, and for increasing libido. The

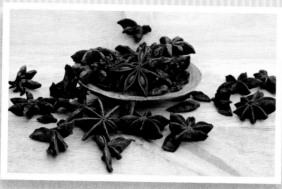

Star anise

essential oil contains shikimic acid, a key ingredient in virus-fighting Tamiflu, and two major antioxidants, linalool and vitamin C. Extracts have treated *Candida albicans*, and in lab tests, four antimicrobial compounds derived from star anise were effective against nearly 70 strains of drug-resistant bacteria.

TURMERIC

Turmeric (*Curcuma longa*) epitomizes the flavors of the Middle East and India—it gives curry its distinct color and taste—while providing valued medicinal benefits. Native to southern Asia, the plant can reach four feet in height and produces large, oval, upright leaves on sturdy stems and spikes of pale pink or white flowers. The spice is processed from the yellow root. For more than 4,500 years, natural healers have relied on this spice to reduce inflammation, fight infection, and ease digestion. It contains curcumin, a powerful antioxidant that purges free radicals. There are indications that curcumin can inhibit certain cancers and may prevent subsequent heart attacks in bypass surgery patients.

VANILLA

This sixteenth-century New World discovery was soon delighting the courts of Europe and has never stopped pleasing dessert lovers. The tropical vanilla orchid vine bears oval green leaves and waxy, delicate, greenish-yellow flowers; these mature into narrow six-inch pod-like fruit with small black seeds. The word *vanilla* comes from the Spanish *vainilla*, meaning "little pod." In pre-Columbian Mexico, it was used to treat indigestion and tension. Today, the flavor compound vanillin is known to reduce cholesterol levels, preventing hardening of the arteries and the formation of blood clots. Its high levels of antioxidants can heal damaged cells, protect the immune system, and diminish the damaging effects of free radicals.

Vanilla

GROW HERBS FOR HEALTH

Herbs are among the easiest plants to grow—provided you have a sunny patch somewhere on your lawn—and can supply you with sweet or savory tastes in the kitchen and a homegrown source of natural medicines.

From the earliest human settlements onward, herbs have been a welcome part of the garden. Primitive cave paintings in France that feature herbs date back to 25,000 BC. During the Middle Ages, herbs appeared in every cottage plot; religious orders in particular grew swaths of sweet-scented or deeply pungent herbs—the former to

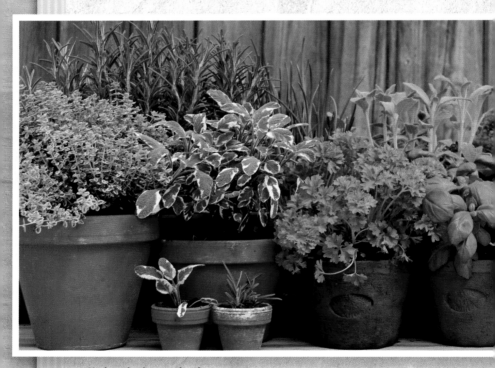

Various herbs growing in pots

nourish their cherished honeybees, the latter to make into rich, ritual incense. By the Victorian era, gardening had reached a zenith, both indoors and out, and wealthy estate owners boasted of conservatories where exotic orchids grew beside collections of rare herbs, while their hardier cousins adorned exterior knot gardens and parterres.

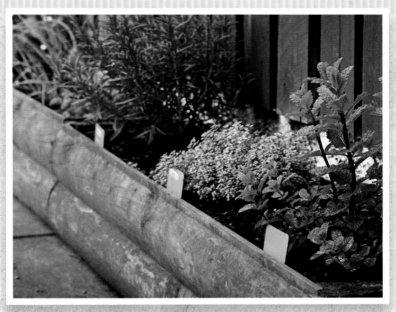

Label your plants with waterproof markers

STEP-BY-STEP

You shouldn't feel the need to create a landscaping masterpiece with your first herb garden, but it pays to follow a few ground rules.

1. Most herbs enjoy the sun, or at least semi-sun. Place your garden where the plants will receive a maximum amount of daylight. Make sure to keep tall varieties such as sage, rosemary, and marjoram at the back, and shorter plants such as parsley and cilantro at the front.

2. If your property is large, consider placing the garden near the house, perhaps as a "kitchen garden" just outside the back door.

3. Before planting, till the soil at least a foot down so that it drains well. Most herbs do not enjoy wet feet. You can improve clay or dense soil with the addition of peat moss, compost, or coarse sand.

4. Starting herbs from seeds can be difficult, so begin with potted plants from a nursery. Dig your holes to twice the width of the root ball.

5. Plant early or late in the day so that delicate baby herbs do not wilt in the hot sun.

6. Space your plants about 18 inches apart; herbs like room to spread out.

7. It's important to label your plants with waterproof markers. The flowers of many herbs look alike, so you won't have them to guide you once the plants enlarge.

GROW HERBS FOR HEALTH

8. If you desire color in your herb garden, plant zinnias, salvia, marigolds, and lantana around the edges. Or create a row of cutting perennials such as coreopsis, day lilies, and rudbeckia, or monarda and echinacea (herbs in their own right).

9. In the beginning, water young plants frequently. Once the plants are established, you can provide a thorough watering a few times a week.

10. You can start harvesting herbs once they mature, taking only a little at a time so that they will quickly replenish their foliage. If you

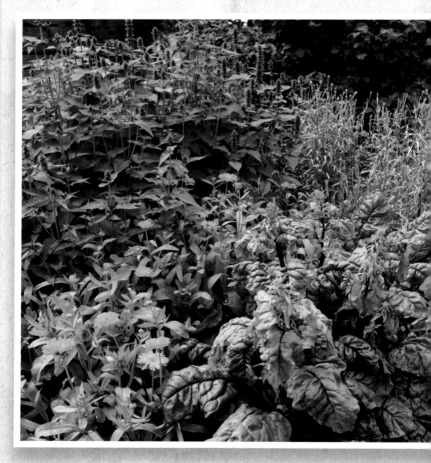

trim more than a third of the plant, their growth will slow. With careful picking, most herbs can be harvested for a few months.

11. Try to pick herbs in the morning, when they are their most flavorful.

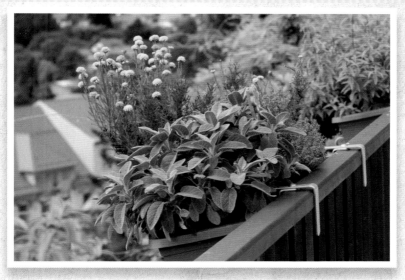

A number of herbs do very well indoors on a sunny windowsill, especially those that feature dwarf varieties. Make sure to keep them misted in winter when home heating dries the air. These herbs include basil ("Greek Miniature"), bay laurel, chervil, chives, dill ("Fern Leaf"), oregano (Greek), parsley (flat leaf), rosemary ("Blue Boy"), sage (dwarf garden), spearmint, and thyme.

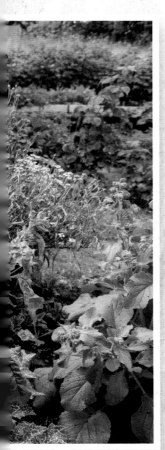

DIY: Suggested Plants

The following herbs are easy to grow and provide a bountiful harvest for eating fresh or drying and preserving. You can plant a striking container with an Italian mix—oregano, basil, and parsley—or a Mexican mix—cilantro, dill, and cayenne peppers.

- basil ("Purple Ruffles" or "Dani")
- sage
- oregano
- dill
- common thyme
- sweet marjoram
- lavender, English or French
- rosemary
- parsley
- chives
- cilantro

DRY OR PRESERVE YOUR OWN HERBS

If your herb garden takes off, and you find yourself with a bumper crop of leafy green produce, never fear. It's simple to dry excess herbs for future culinary use—or to make your own decorative sachets, potpourris, or wreaths.

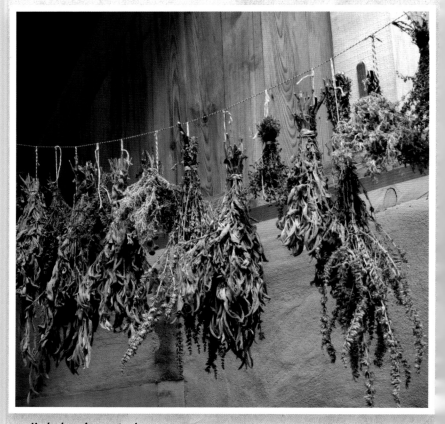

Herbs hanging up to dry

THE BASIC HOW-TOS

Most people who grow herbs find some occasion to dry them, and there are a number of techniques that work well. Your ultimate goal is for the herbs to dry out without any trace of moisture, mold, or mildew. You also want the maximum flavor retention. Most dried herbs gain potency, while a few others lose it. You will also discover that "fresh" dried herbs beat out their packaged, store-bought cousins in terms of taste, intensity, and aroma.

Hang Ups: The simplest solution for preserving herbs is copying what humans have done for millennia: hanging them up to dry. Tie your herbs into small bundles using twist ties so you can tighten them as the stems shrink. Place muslin or a mesh or brown bag with a few holes in it around the bundle and fasten it at the top. Any warm dry place that is not your kitchen should work as a location. Once the herbs are properly dried—they're brittle to the touch and crumble easily—it's time to store them in sealed glass containers. You may be inclined to grind them all first, but intact herbs maintain their character far longer than ground ones.

Solar Dehydrator: These drying frames can be easily made by stapling mesh screening onto two large flat frames and placing your herbs between the layers. The sun will do all the work after you lay them out on a deck or porch until the herbs are withered. You can also buy round, tiered hanging mesh racks online.

Oven Warming: This method takes time and effort. The herbs need to be dried at 100°F, and require air circulation, which is difficult to achieve in ventless ovens. Arrange the herbs on a cheesecloth-covered cooling rack and watch over them as they dry. Microwaves can also dry herbs, but they too need constant attention. Strip leaves off stems and place them between two paper towels. Start with one minute on high, then rest for 30 seconds. Then alternate 30 seconds on, 30 off, until the herbs are the right consistency. It may take 10 minutes.

The Neglect Method: Most of us have discovered this method by accident. We collected a bunch of herbs, put them on a table or counter, then forget they were there for a week or two. We ended up with nicely dried herbs, unless they got moldy or were nibbled on by mice. Still, this method does work if you're willing to accept less-than-stellar results. Another easy trick is leaving herbs outside their packaging in a refrigerator; they will often end up crisp, colorful, and flavorful.

DIY: Herbal Door Wreath

To create this beautiful home ornament you will need a willow or Styrofoam form, some florist's wire, and a pair of strong scissors or shears, plus a collection of dried aromatic herbs. Begin by placing a bundle of the same herbs on the wreath and securing it with wire; move to the next section and add a different bundle, trying to vary the shapes and textures of the herbs. Continue around the entire wreath, aiming for a pleasant, consistent fullness. If any wires are exposed, tuck in single stems to obscure them or augment with dried baby's breath. Add a wire hanger at the back and adorn with a simple raffia bow.

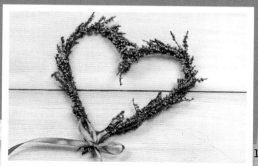

HEALTHFUL STORES & SOURCES

When you feel the onset of illness or get that urge to improve the quality of your life, where can you turn to find the herbs, healing plants, and supplements you require to make those healthy new choices?

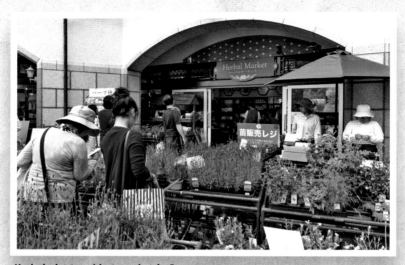

Herbal plants sold at market in Japan

You've heard all the buzzwords—whole foods, organic crops, farm-to-table movement—and now you're determined to follow a better diet, including all those nutritious, antioxidant herbs. Fortunately, we live in an era of instant gratification. If you are suddenly transfixed with the notion of a healthier body, you can go online and find almost any herb or natural supplement you've read about and order it in quantity. But that's only part of the equation. When you are starting out on a new journey, it's important to have a roadmap, and the same goes for any expeditions into natural, healing foods. You will need a knowledgeable guide, someone who can initiate you into the language and customs. That person is the proprietor of a health-food or natural-foods store.

HEALTH-FOOD STORES
Unlike the clerks in most other stores, health-food store managers understand that part of their job is guiding newbies through the sometimes-confusing world of herbal supplements and alternative medicines. They will not only help you choose a remedy for an existing

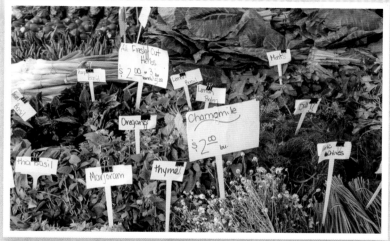

Herb stand at a local farmers market in Richmond, Virginia

ailment, they can show you an array of herbs that boost immunity and help keep diseases at bay. These stores also carry organic foods, local produce, environmentally conscious products, and special-needs diet items, and should have a stock of essential oils, distilled from herbs and other botanicals, that can be used medicinally, as aromatherapy, or simply as enlivening scents.

ASIAN GROCERIES

These large, vegetable market–type stores can be goldmines for locating fresh herbs, hard-to-find dried herbs, and healing spices. And their prices are usually quite competitive. Try Japanese markets for sampling different types of beneficial seaweed and algae or Korean markets for gut-healthy fermented kimchi. Indian markets offer their own blends of masala, curry, or chai spices, and stock exotic teas.

SPECIALTY SHOPS

These are the gourmet groceries that specialize in hard-to-find items and artisanal breads, beverages, and dishes. They are ideal for finding unusual culinary herbs or spices that you might require for medicinal purposes. Look for vanilla beans and saffron—you may pay a premium but you will be getting the real thing.

HEALTH FOOD LINGO

Superfood: Any food that offers high levels of vitamins, minerals, and phytochemicals. Most fruits, vegetables, and herbs fit this definition.

Organic: Produce grown without manmade pesticides, fertilizers, or GMOs, and livestock raised without unnecessary chemicals, medications, feed additives, or growth hormones.

Probiotic: The term indicates that a food replenishes the natural, healthy fauna in the gut.

Fermentation: When the sugar in a food or beverage has been broken down by the presence of yeast or bacteria.

Gluten free: Foods that contain no gluten, a mixture of proteins found in wheat and some other grains. Gluten-free foods include rice, cassava, soy, corn, potato, tapioca, beans, sourghum, spelt, amaranth, and buckwheat.

HERBAL CURES

Who has not suffered through a bad cold or cough? Or been laid low with a bout of the flu? Respiratory issues should not be taken lightly, so be sure to treat them at the first sign of a sniffle.

Many herbal remedies for colds, coughs, and sore throats go back thousands of years. This does not mean they are less effective than modern medications—many of them were the source for over-the-counter aids such as horehound cough drops and mentholated rubs.

COLDS AND FLU

Colds and flus are viral infections of the upper respiratory system that affect the nose, sinuses, upper airways, throat, windpipe, and bronchi. Symptoms include sneezing, wheezing, coughing, a runny nose and eyes, and congestion. Bear in mind that because these ailments are viral, they do not respond to antibiotics; the best course is to treat the symptoms.

Supplements: If you fear a cold is looming, it's wise to take herbal and vitamin supplements to boost your immune system and shorten the cold's duration. These can include versatile nettle leaf, time-tested herbs such as echinacea and ginseng, decongestant ginger, nutritionally essential zinc, antioxidant vitamin C, immunity boosting vitamins A and D, crushed raw garlic, antibacterial and antiviral oil of oregano, virus-battling circumin, bee-produced propolis, and fever-reducing white willow bark.

Elderberry Elixir: This traditional syrup recipe provides phytonutrient benefits to ease inflammation and clear congestion, especially during the flu.

Recipe: Combine half a cup of black elderberries (other colors are toxic) with 3 cups of water and simmer for 30 minutes. Strain into a container and add a cup of honey to the cooled syrup. Take a tablespoon every 4 hours to treat a cold or flu. A sealed, refrigerated container will keep for 3 months.

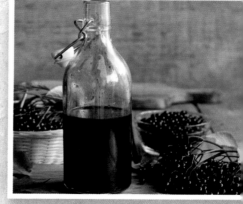

Elderberry syrup is a powerful curative

Hot Ginger Tea: Hot drinks are crucial for colds because they furnish fluids and steaming vapors that can break up congestion. This spicy, warming beverage will ease a scratchy throat, reduce swelling of the mucous membranes, and loosen phlegm.

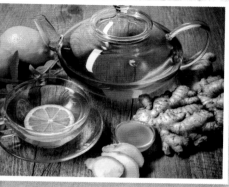

Healing ginger tea

Recipe: Pour 4 cups of boiling water over 6 to 8 tablespoons of grated ginger root in a glass jar. Add a pinch of cinnamon, a squirt of lemon juice, and a teaspoon of honey. Cover the jar and let the mixture steep for 45 minutes, then strain and drink. Keep the remainder in refrigerator for 1 day.

Epsom Salt Bath: A hot soak in salts—perhaps with the addition of mint or eucalyptus oil—will restore any depleted magnesium, which is essential to your immune system, and will help clear your sinuses and relieve your muscle aches.

Quick Tips: Try adding lemon juice to sage tea. Use eucalyptus oil rubs to open swollen passages. Boil cardamom with cinnamon in a few cups of water and gargle to relieve sore throats. Mix cayenne pepper with lemon juice and honey in a cup of hot water and drink daily for a natural decongestant.

COUGHS

Even after colds diminish, coughing and hoarseness caused by post-nasal drip can linger. Gargling with warm water can help, but you can also curb the symptoms with natural soothers and tonics.

Honey Combos: Honey, which bees produce from flower nectar, is a natural antiseptic and can soothe even the sorest throat. Swallow a teaspoonful for a sweet remedy, or try adding 2 teaspoons to herbal teas, heated water and lemon juice, or hot oatmeal, or drizzling it over French toast.

Mullein Tea: When dried, this common wildflower of roadsides and open fields makes an effective expectorant by thinning phlegm so it can be coughed up.
Recipe: Combine 2 tablespoons dried mullein with 2 or 3 teaspoons dried thyme (another natural expectorant) in a large mug and pour 1 ½ cups boiling water over the herbs. Stir, let it steep, then strain and add honey or lemon to taste. Drink twice daily to ease congestion.

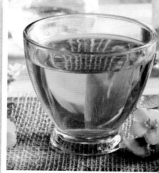

Mullein tea

SEASONAL ALLERGIES

People who suffer from seasonal allergies such as hay fever or allergic rhinitis are frequently plagued with the sneezing, itchy eyes, sinus pressure, headaches, and chest congestion that can make life a misery for several months each year.

COMBAT ALLERGIES NATURALLY

Allergies are the immune system's reaction or hypersensitivity to an antigen, an "exaggerated or pathological immunological response" to a substance or physical state. Irritants can include pollen, dust, dust mites, animal fur or dander, or certain foods. Although there are plenty of over-the-counter allergy medications—decongestants, cough suppressants, sinus treatments, and antihistamines—most of them come with a long list of side effects: drowsiness, dizziness, palpitations, dry eyes, or severe dry mouth. Why not turn to some of the time-tested allergy remedies favored by the natural-medicine community? They can help you combat the effects of congestion and histamines—the substances triggered as allergic responses when dust or pollen come into contact with mucus membranes—with few or no side effects.

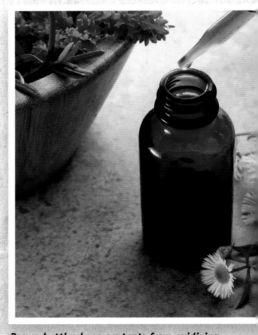

Brown bottles keep contents from oxidizing

Stinging Nettle Therapy:

This long-valued herb, a common wildflower that grows worldwide, may actually be a natural antihistamine. In allergy studies, nearly 60 percent of the participants who took a daily dose of 300 mg of freeze-dried nettles found their symptoms cleared. Stinging nettles can be purchased at health-food stores or online.

The Quercetin Effect: This powerful antioxidant flavonoid, which provided antihistamine effects in lab studies, can be found in ginkgo biloba, Saint-John's-wort, green tea, berries, apples, oranges, grapes, onions, buckwheat, and olive oil. Quercetin also prevents free radicals, supports heart health, and reduces pain and inflammation.

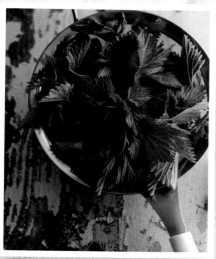

Stinging nettle therapy

Bromelain Benefits: This enzyme, which is found in pineapples or in supplements, has the ability to reduce swelling or inflammation in the nasal passages and sinuses. It can reduce the symptoms of asthma, which can be allergy related, and it also promotes digestion, wound healing, and relief of body aches. Studies indicate that the optimum dose is 400–500 mg three times a day.

The Vitamin C Option: Ascorbic acid is yet another natural antihistamine; it is found in many fruits and vegetables or can be taken as a supplement. It can help you treat a stuffy nose or scratchy throat with no side effects. The recommended dosage for blocking antihistamines is a minimum of 2 grams a day; or eat several oranges or grapefruit daily.

Quick Tips: Try sipping a cup of water with a teaspoon of apple cider vinegar and a squirt of lemon juice. Taking a tablespoon of raw honey daily will help you increase tolerance for the local pollen that is causing your reactions. Eat crushed garlic or garlic supplements. Inhale eucalyptus or frankincense oil.

DIY: The Neti Pot

This small "teapot" allows you to pour warm water up one nostril until it fills your nasal passages and drains out the other nostril. Although it sounds painful, the concept of flushing the sinuses is a painless part of traditional yoga. The practice can noticably improve chronic sinus sufferers, those with severe allergies, and people recovering from a cold. It's best to use distilled water or boiled water warmed to a comfortable temperature.

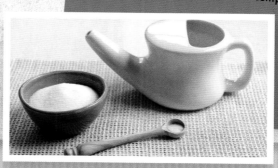

Neti pot

URINARY AND BLADDER PROBLEMS

Few complaints are as uncomfortable as a urinary tract infection, with its pain, cramping, and frequent need to visit the bathroom. Although women get more bladder infections, men are more prone to highly painful kidney stones.

The urinary tract consists of two kidneys, two ureters, the bladder, and the urethra. The kidneys' job is to maintain fluid balance as well as filter waste from blood and process it into urine. Urine is then passed through the ureters to the bladder for storage, before flowing through the urethra and out of the body. A number of ailments affect this tract, some of them treatable at home. When a more serious issue is suspected, a urologist performs as cystoscopy, inserting a thin tube with a tiny camera into the urethra and up into the bladder. Many kidney problems can be diagnosed with blood tests or an ultrasound.

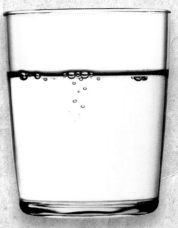

Drink plenty of water

URINARY TRACT INFECTIONS

UTIs occur when bacteria enter the body through the urethra and travel into the bladder, where they multiply. Female anatomy is often the reason women get more urinary tract infections—either E. coli from the anus touches the urethra or other contaminants are introduced during vaginal sex. Symptoms include burning pain during urination; frequency, or the sensation of needing to pee after urination; and urgency, or a fierce need to pee that sends you racing for the bathroom.

Water Method: The primary treatment is drinking 8 to 12 glasses of water a day to flush out bacteria.

Berry Remedy: Try drinking 3 cups of cranberry juice or eating half a cup of blueberries—they both reduce the number of bacteria clinging to the urethra. Juniper berries act as a diuretic and can also flush out urinary bacteria and toxins.

Baking Soda Solution: Lower the acidity of your urine by mixing one tablespoon of baking soda in a cup of water and drinking it each morning for a week.

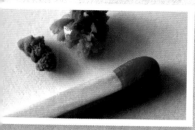

Kidney stones compared to the head of a matchstick

KIDNEY STONES

These small, hard deposits occur when minerals and salts, such as calcium oxilate, crystallize in the kidneys and must pass out through the urinary tract. Chronic dehydration is one cause, weight gain is another. Symptoms include pain in the side and back, pain that radiates to the groin, and spasmodic cramping. One proven remedy is fluid therapy: drinking enough liquids to help flush the small stones. Larger stones may need medical intervention.

Lemon Juice: Lemon juice, which can break down mineral deposits, may actually reduce the size of the stones. Drink 5 ounces of fresh lemon juice in the morning and another 5 ounces just before dinner.

Basil Extract: Basil can prevent stones from forming by stabilizing uric acid levels. Take one teaspoon of basic extract or juice daily. The herb's acetic acid can break down stones. Apple cider vinegar contains citric acid, which also dissolves calcium deposits. Try 2 tablespoons in a cup of water to ease the pain and prevent stones from occurring.

Wheatgrass Washout: This herb contains compounds that stimulate urine production, helping the stones to pass less painfully. Take 2 to 8 ounces of extract daily, or use supplements or pills. Celery juice and celery seed both have similar effects.

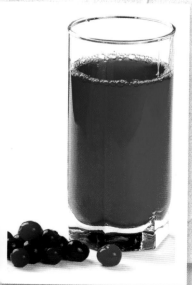

Bean Broth: A broth made from kidney beans will supply high amounts of magnesium, a mineral that both shrinks the stones and eases the symptoms. Remove the beans from their pods, simmer them for 5 to 6 hours, strain, and serve. The broth should be taken at least twice a day.

Quick tips: Other treatments for relieving kidney stones are dandelion extract, pomegranate or aloe juice, and chamomile or peppermint tea.

TREATING THE UPPER GI TRACT

Gastric distress may consist of gas, heartburn, indigestion, bloating, nausea, and cramping, which make it hard to focus on anything but your discomfort and embarrassment. Fortunately, many herbal remedies can offer speedy relief.

The upper gastrointestinal tract is made up of the mouth; pharynx; esophagus; the bean-shaped stomach, where acid and enzymes handle the majority of digestion; and the duodenum, the top of the small intestine. This group of organs can suffer from easy-to-treat conditions such as indigestion and gas, or more problematic issues such as acid reflux, ulcers, or cancer. Maintaining a healthy diet, including lots of fiber and nutrients, is one way to keep the upper GI tract relatively trouble free.

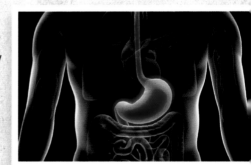

The stomach

INDIGESTION

Indigestion, or dyspepsia, is a persistant pain or discomfort in the upper abdomen caused by poor digestion. Symptoms include gassiness, heartburn, bloating, and nausea. Causes include overeating, allergies, gastritis (inflammation of the stomach lining), nerves, stress, GERD, pregnancy, or food poisoning.

Herbal Assists: Antispasmodic and anti-inflammatory chamomile tea eliminates gas and bloating; ginger aids digestion, eases intestinal muscles, and relieves gas. Coriander's digestive properties can settle the stomach; for a soothing tea, add a teaspoon of dried coriander leaves to a cup of hot water. Garlic is a natural anti-inflammatory and antibiotic that can turn off the fire of heartburn. Peppermint contains antispasmodic menthol oil that calms the tummy and reduces spasms.

Pantry Helpers: Apple cider vinegar promotes digestion; steamed or boiled pumpkin is full of antioxidants that can relieve gas and stomach pain, as well as nutrients such as vitamin A, fiber, and potassium that ease indigestion.

Spice Solutions: Caraway seeds are antispasmodic and antimicrobial; they relax the stomach muscles and trigger the expulsion of gas. Fennel seeds are effective digestives that can counteract bloating. Black pepper stimulates the gastric flow of hydrochloric acid to improve sluggish digestion.

ACID REFLUX

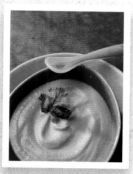

Also called GERD—for "gastroesophageal reflux disease"—this condition occurs when the sphincter between the esophagus and stomach allows digestive acid to splash into the gullet. Symptoms may be a burning sensation or the taste of stomach contents rising in the throat. The resulting pain and pressure can feel like a heart attack. GERD may require a doctor's care, but there are ways to ease the burning sensation. Avoiding food triggers and eating smaller meals are good first steps.

Pureed pumpkin

Cool it Down: Turmeric coats the lining of the GI tract and prevents stomach acid from rising. Drinking aloe vera juice has become increasingly popular with GERD sufferers. Digestive enzyme supplements can help, as can taking a tablespoon of apple cider vinegar in a cup of water before meals.

GASTRITIS

This is a group of conditions that inflame the stomach lining, resulting in burning, nausea, and pain. It can be caused by a lack of vitamin B-12, overuse of anti-inflammatory painkillers, or, most commonly, *Helicobacter pylori*, a bacteria that also produces stomach ulcers. Begin the healing process by reducing stress and eating lighter meals.

Gut Reactions: Although *H. pylori* requires treatment with antibiotics, there are natural remedies that will help reduce the symptoms of gastritis. Try taking a garlic extract supplement; add probiotics to your diet; neutralize stomach acid with baking soda in water; and drink ginger, peppermint, chamomile or antioxidant green tea. Avoid alcohol and spicy foods, and eat strawberries, which can prevent the inflammation from occurring.

DIY: Probiotics

Although some skeptics scoff, many health-conscious people regularly add these living microorganisms—bacteria and yeasts—to their diet to improve health, aid digestion, and prevent or treat certain illnesses. Probiotics are found in cultured or fermented foods such as yogurt, kefir, kimchi, sauerkraut, tempeh, miso, and pickles, as well as in supplements.

HELP FOR THE LOWER GI TRACT

The lower gastrointestinal tract is prone to a number of problems—constipation, diarrhea, painful bloating—that can put a cramp in your day. Yet these can be easily treated with natural remedies and healing tonics.

The lower part of the digestive tract begins with the small intestine, where food breaks down into nutrients that are absorbed; the large intestine or colon, where waste is processed; and the anus, through which stool is then eliminated. The remaining water in the large intestine returns to the bloodstream. Serious or chronic diseases of the lower GI need a doctor's care, but many ailments can be treated at home.

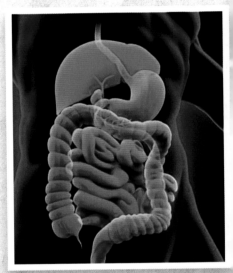

The intestines

CONSTIPATION

If you have fewer than three bowel movement a week, you may be constipated. This can be caused by a fast-food diet that is high fat, low fiber; lack of hydration or exercise; medications; or anxiety. Symptoms are typically a hard, dry stool or movements that are difficult or even painful to expel. Ignoring the condition only makes it worse. Start the healing process by drinking more water, upping your intake of fiber, starting on probiotics, and exercising lightly.

Herbal Helpers: Drink aloe vera juice, a natural laxative; take constipation-relieving supplements such as slippery elm, fenugreek seeds, nettle, dandelion, sorrel, or sea buckthorn. Add oily sesame seeds to salads or hot dishes; drink mint or ginger tea.

Pantry Picks: Drink a cup of hot water with a spoonful of honey or lemon juice, or both; add high-fiber dried fruit to your diet; take a tablespoon of blackstrap molasses at bedtime.

DIARRHEA

A bout of diarrhea—loose, watery stool with cramping, bloating, and gas—can make for a very uncomfortable few days. It is often caused by an intestinal virus, food poisoning (if you suspect this is the case, call your doctor), allergies, medications, diabetes, or alcohol abuse. It is probably one of the first ailments early humans sought to treat—because there was no refrigeration—and so there are many effective herbal fixes. Begin by drinking lots of fluids to replenish your electrolytes.

Herbal Remedies: Drink decaffeinated black tea or blackberry, raspberry, or chamomile herbal tea to calm intestinal inflammation; dice the skin of an organic orange, steep it in hot water, and strain, then add honey to taste. Ground psyllium makes stool bulkier—take one to three teaspoons in water daily. Ayurvedic healers advise taking half a teaspoon of ginger in a cup of buttermilk three times a day.

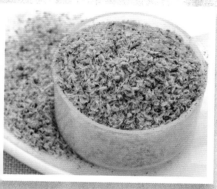

Psyllium-seed husks

Kitchen Aids: Rice has a naturally binding effect on the bowel. If you suspect a bacterial infection, sip apple cider vinegar in a cup of water; its pectin content will also calm spasms. Eating a quarter cup of pureed pumpkin or carrot per hour is quite effective.

IRRITABLE BOWEL SYNDROME

IBS is a chronic condition that afflicts the large intestine with cramping, gas, constipation, and diarrhea. Onset of episodes can be sudden, so planned activities end up iffy at best. It can be managed with changes in diet, lifestyle, and attitude. Eliminating dairy and fat-heavy dishes also works for many sufferers. Begin recovery by eating smaller meals and increasing fiber.

Healing Herbs: Licorice root tea is known to relieve irritation of the bowel. Peppermint, taken as tea or capsules, can eliminate most symptoms. Aloe vera juice and chamomile tea are both beneficial.

DIY: Replenish Electrolytes

It's easy to mix up your own electrolyte-boosting beverage by combining ½ cup orange juice; ¼ cup lemon juice; 2 cups water, green tea, or coconut water; 2 tablespoons raw honey or maple syrup; and ⅛ teaspoon quality salt.

FEMALE REPRODUCTIVE HEALTH

For centuries, many of women's legitimate reproductive concerns were chalked up to "hysteria" by the medical professions. Today, woman control their own health decisions, and many of them choose natural or herbal options.

The female reproductive system—the vagina, cervix, uterus, and ovaries—prepares itself for a possible pregnancy nearly every month from the onset of puberty until menopause. This results in a series of conflicting, hormone-based emotions and often-painful physical symptoms that women experience over and over for decades. The reproductive system is also susceptible to endometriosis, when uterine tissue forms in the abdominal cavity, and benign uterine tumors called fibroids. It is at risk from sexually transmitted diseases, such as syphilis or HIV/AIDS, and invasive cancers. Many of these problems require medical treatment, but some conditions can be addressed with natural healing.

Rou Gui

MENSTRUATION
Many women experience normal periods, but occasionally they are accompanied by painful cramping, called dysmenorrhea. Other problems may include nausea, migraines, irregular cycles, and heavy flow. There is also PMS, premenstrual syndrome, which appears prior to the period, and can cause bloating, irritability, headaches, insomnia, and cravings.

Cramp Relief: Women with cramps can turn to antispasmodic blue cohosh in conjunction with black cohosh, which contains isoflavones that affect estrogen levels. A traditional Chinese tea called Rou Gui

132

is another remedy; it's prepared with medicinal cinnamon. Other effective herbs include chaste tree berry, bilberry, evening primrose, and feverfew. Dong quai, a Chinese herb high in vitamin B-12, will relax cramps and treat PMS and menopause. In fact, most herbs that ease cramps also help PMS. Other effective PMS remedies are lemon balm, burdock, Saint-John's-wort, and ginkgo.

VAGINAL HEALTH

The vagina is a marvelous, complex organ, but it also faces a continuous threat of contamination from the anus and urethra. Sexual activity without protection against STDs furnishes another risk. And because the organ's interior is not visible, many women remain unaware of a problem until there is pain or a discharge. The most common vaginal ailments are yeast infections caused by *Candida albicans*. They result in itching, burning, redness, irritation, and dryness. Start recovery by keeping the area scrupulously clean and wearing soft cotton clothing.

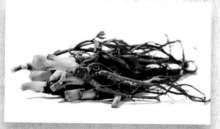

Dong quai

Replace the Fauna: Just as in the gut, the moist interior of the vagina contains beneficial bacteria, such as *Lactobacillus acidophilus. Candida* can seriously deplete them, so make sure you are taking probiotics and eating fermented foods. For itching, prepare a douche using 2 tablespoons of apple cider vinegar in a cup of water, and for dryness try natural lubricants such as jojoba oil, aloe, or vitamin E. Other remedies for vaginal infections include elderberry, milk thistle, boric acid, vitamin C, and the essential oils of tea tree, lavender, and myrrh.

MENOPAUSE:

Although this signals the surcease of their periods, many women find it the most difficult part of the menses process. In addition to the emotional issues related to loss of fertility, they face lowered libido, painful intercourse, vaginal itching, mood swings, hot flashes, and palpitations.

Find Balance: In ayurvedic medicine, ashwagandha is used to relieve hot flashes and anxiety; maca root, or Peruvian ginseng, can improve lack of libido, hot flashes, and night sweats. Chinese dong quai helps to maintain and balance female hormones, as does black cohosh, which also reduces vaginal dryness and hot flashes. Vitamin E can also eliminate hot flashes.

MALE REPRODUCTIVE PROBLEMS

Men may potentially face a number of reproductive issues, including impotence, loss of libido, and prostate problems. The use of some common herbs— and some exotic ones as well—can help improve both performance and reproductive health.

The male reproductive system is comprised of the testicles, which produce sperm and testosterone; the penis, which ejaculates semen; and the prostate gland, which secretes a fluid that nourishes the sperm and is released as semen. A urologist oversees any disorders concerning the function of these organs, but medical treatments for sexual impotence or infertility can be augmented with herbal remedies, as can some benign prostate concerns.

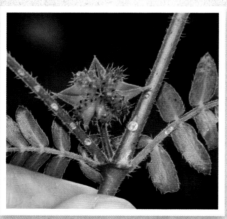

Tribulus terrestris

IMPOTENCE
Decreased sexual function or lowered libido in men may be caused by age, disease, medications, stress, or emotional issues. A number of herbal supplements have a long history of successfully addressing these problems, but should be discussed with a physician prior to inclusion in a treatment plan.

Return of Vigor: In a clinical study, an ayurvedic herb called *Tribulus terrestris L.* was effective for increasing sexual desire and enhancing erections. It may work by increasing levels of a male hormone, DHEA. Another exotic herb found in Arabic medicine is ferula asafoetida. In a group study its extracts were able to revive libido and potency in 60 percent of participating men. Red ginseng contains the active compound saponin, which may account for its long history of restoring sexual desire and vigor and increasing patient satisfaction. Ginkgo biloba is known as a brain booster, but it may also help alleviate the sexual dysfunction often caused by antidepressant medications.

INFERTILITY

It's a delicate matter, determining who is at fault when a couple cannot conceive. In one in five couples, the man is the culprit. One in twenty men has a low sperm count, a surprising one in a hundred men has no sperm in his semen. This could be due to lack of production or to poor transport. Other issues that affect fertility may be the inability to maintain an erection, a blockage between the testes and penis, low levels of pituitary hormones, or sperm antibodies.

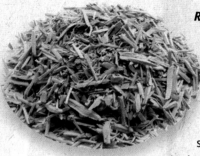

Natural Viagra, muira puama

Restore Virility: Aside from recommended physical accommodations—avoiding hot baths, tight underwear, and alcohol—men with low sperm counts can combat free radicals, which can damage sperm, by increasing their intake of supplements that contain antioxidants, especially beta-carotenes such as vitamins A, C, and E, and selenium and zinc. Herbal supplements such as saw palmetto, muira puama, ginkgo biloba, and *Rhodiola rosea* should be taken for at least three months—the time it takes sperm to form.

PROSTATE HEALTH

As men age, their prostate glands may become enlarged, causing urinary issues. These can include urgency, frequency, difficulty voiding, burning, and leakage. Medical intervention often requires medication that may help to shrink the prostate, while saw palmetto berry

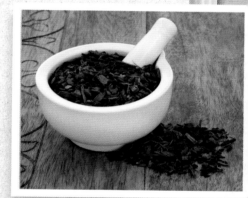

Pygeum bark herb

extract can reduce prostate size by altering certain hormone levels. An effective tea can be made by pouring a pint of boiling water over 1/8 cup of watermelon seeds and letting it steep before straining and drinking. Other proven aids include stinging nettle, African plum tree bark (pygeum), garlic extract, and the multi-herb remedy beta-sitosterol.

DIY: The Facilitators

Men who suffer from erectile dysfunction often have low levels of dehydroepiandrosterone (DHEA), a natural adrenal hormone that converts to both estrogen and testosterone. Fortunately, there are effective DHEA supplements made from wild yam extract and soy. L-arginine supplements mimic an amino acid that helps to make nitric oxide, which relaxes blood vessels and allows an easier erection

CARDIOVASCULAR HEALTH

The heart and its interconnected blood vessels—arteries, veins, and capillaries—comprise the circulatory system, an amazing network that is capable of sending five liters of blood through it every single minute.

The hardworking heart muscle drives the cardiovascular system, which makes sure oxygen, nutrients, hormones, and cellular waste products reach the proper parts of the body. The system can be affected by circulatory issues—among them hardening of the arteries, high cholesterol, blood-pressure problems, or stroke, as well as blood diseases and heart conditions, such as coronary disease, which imperils the heart's arteries and is the top killer of adult men and women in the United States. Preventative measures are always preferred to surgical solutions, and botanicals offer many properties that can heal, strengthen, and maintain the cardiovascular network.

HEART-HEALTHY OPTIONS

Herbs and spices can offer many forms of assistance to the circulatory system, from lowering cholesterol, blood pressure, and blood sugar, to thinning the blood and steadying heartbeat, to avoiding strokes, to acting as a healing tonic for the heart itself.

Lower Those Levels: Garlic (and its cousin, the onion) has a long history of lowering cholesterol and to some extent blood pressure, treating arteriosclerosis, and preventing stroke that goes back to Stone Age laborers and the builders of the pyramids. These beneficial effects are believed to be the result of the plant's sulfur-bearing compounds. Anti-inflammatory ginger can thin the blood, reduce bad cholesterol, and relax the blood vessels, which lowers blood pressure. Green tea, with its many

Onions and garlic

DIY: A Sweet Cure

Cinnamon helps to prevent heart disease by inhibiting the release of fatty acids, which then reduces the inflammation of platelet membranes in the blood, thus keeping it at the proper viscosity. This can subsequently lower blood pressure. This spice also lowers bad cholesterol and harmful triglycerides. Add half a teaspoon of this tangy spice to your morning tea or coffee or sprinkle some on your hot cereal.

antioxidants and flavonoids, is another go-to for its ability to strength the lining of the heart and blood vessels, while battling triglycerides and bad cholesterol.

Boost Heart Function: Hawthorn (*Crataegus oxycanthus*) had a long history in the natural-healing community as the go-to herb for increasing the strength of the heart, and in the 1800s medical doctors began experimenting with the herb, with encouraging results. The leaves, flowers, and fruit all contain chemical compounds that increase blood flow, and can treat angina pectoris, arrhythmia, and circulatory insufficiency in addition to heart disease. Hawthorn is safe for long-term use and should be taken for several months to be truly effective. Motherwort (*Leonurus cardiaca*) is another respected tonic that benefits the circulatory system; this herb has been used to strengthen the heart and treat palpitations, mild irregularities, and high blood pressure. It too should be taken for a period of several months.

Bring the Heat: Cayenne pepper and its active ingredient, capsaicin, are known to fight free radicals, prevent blood clots, and dilate blood vessels, which lowers blood pressure. The herb also increases metabolism and helps with weight loss, two other factors in maintaining a healthy ticker.

Cardio Champs: Other powerhouse herbs that impact the heart include turmeric, with its circulation-stimulating curcumin; thyme, which combats free radicals that can damage the cardiovascular system; antioxidant cardamom, which lowers blood pressure; cardioprotective fenugreek seeds; and coriander, with its antioxidant and antiplatelet compounds; it also helps to manage diabetes, a risk factor for heart disease. Tasty hibiscus tea can reduce hardening of the arteries and high blood pressure.

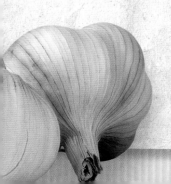

Cinnamon

ENDOCRINE ISSUES

The endocrine system consists of a network of interconnected glands that oversee the heartbeat, how bones and tissues grow, the conversion of food into calories that fuel our bodies, metabolism, immunity, and sexual reproduction.

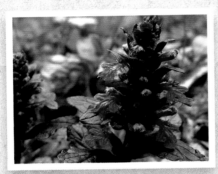

Bugleweed

This system includes the pituitary or "master gland," which sits at the base of the brain and influences other glands; the adrenals, atop the kidneys, which secrete the hormone cortisol; the thyroid in the throat, which controls metabolism; the islet cells of the pancreas, which release the hormones glycogen and insulin; the thymus in the upper chest, which affects immunity; and the ovaries and testes, which facilitate reproduction. The pineal gland in the brain is linked to sleep patterns, while the hypothalamus in the middle brain talks to the pituitary. Any disruption of one gland can affect one or more of the others, resulting in an imbalance that may require the care of an endocrinologist. Still, there are natural methods for keeping these systems healthy and doing their critical jobs.

COPING WITH DIABETES

When carbohydrates in the body are not metabolized properly due to an impaired response to the hormone insulin, glucose levels in blood and urine can elevate dangerously. This condition is known as diabetes. Type 1 begins in childhood; it is quite serious and requires injections of insulin. Type 2 occurs as people age; it can be treated with pills and dietary alterations, as well as herbal remedies that help stabilize glucose levels in the body.

Find the Balance: In addition to a low-fat, high-fiber diet, diabetics can turn to mineral supplements such as magnesium, potassium, zinc, and chromium picolinate, and to antidiabetics such as aloe vera, cinnamon, ginseng, ginger, dandelion root, ginkgo biloba, alfalfa, and stinging nettle. Blueberry and huckleberry help increase insulin production; the Indian drug called gymnena sylvestre ("sugar destroyer" in Hindi) lowers blood sugar; evening primrose oil contains GLA, gamma-linolenic acid, which may be lacking in diabetics; bitter melon supplements block sugar absorption in the intestines; bilberry contains anthocyanidins that prevent diabetic damage to tiny blood vessels; and fenugreek lowers blood sugar and bad cholesterol.

THYROID PROBLEMS

When this butterfly-shaped gland overproduces hormones, a condition called hyperthyroidism, people become sluggish, fatigued, and depressed. Hyperthyroidism, or overproduction, results in anxiety, sweating, insomnia, and weight issues. A benign growth on the gland is called a goiter and can result in either of the above conditions.

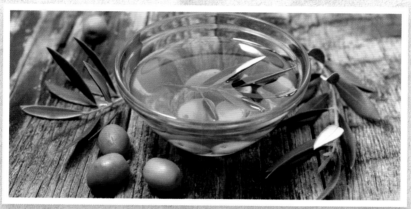

Olive oil

Healthy Remedies: Underproduction by the thyroid can be addressed by lemon balm, bugleweed, verbena, B vitamins, and selenium. Treat overproduction with green smoothies, and anti-inflammatory herbs such as rosemary, basil, oregano, and kelp. Ashwaganda is beneficial to both the thyroid and the adrenals and is adaptogenic, meaning it can help adapt to and deal with stress. Other adaptogens include holy basil, ginseng, and licorice root. Frankincense and myrrh also ease stress and improve thyroid function. Proteolytic enzymes such as the bromelain found in pineapples can reduce thyroid inflammation.

ADRENAL CRISIS

Adrenal insufficiency—which results in chronic fatigue, weight loss, and depression—may occur when these glands do not produce enough cortisol, the hormone that regulates stress. A buildup of stress or an autoimmune reaction can eventually result in a severe hormonal imbalance.

Regain Vitality: First increase intake of healthy fats such as coconut and olive oils, leafy greens, and fish with omega-3 fatty acids. Next make a real effort to reduce stress levels. Then consider supplements such as licorice root and magnesium, and adaptogens such as ashwagandha and holy basil.

PREVENTATIVE FOOT CARE

Mobility is the key to staying fit through middle age and into the senior years. That means foot care and foot health are important to men and woman at almost any age; they are especially critical for diabetics.

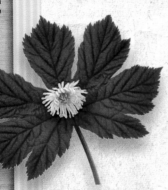

Goldenseal

As a species that walks upright, humans put a lot of pressure on their feet. Overpronation—rolling the foot to one side—can lead to hammer toes, arch pain, arthritis, and Achilles tendonitis. Keeping feet confined in sweaty, narrow shoes, especially those with high heels, results in bunions, calluses, corns, ingrown toenails, and fungal infections. Those high heels are why women experience four times as many foot issues as men.

BUNIONS

These inflamed, bony bumps, called hallux valgus, form on the joint at the base of the big toe. They occur when the big toe pushes against the next toe, forcing the big toe's joint to expand. Bunions are possibly genetic or may be caused by arthritis or tight, pointy shoes. If the little toe is affected it is called a bunionette or tailor's bunion.

Foot Massage: Soothe bunions with a massage of warm olive, castor, or coconut oil. Turmeric, with its pain-blocking qualities, can be mixed with oil and rubbed in or taken topically. Bathing the foot in Epsom salts will lessen the pain, and the magnesium in the salt should reduce swelling. A similar bath can also soften ingrown toenails; afterward, gently push swollen skin away from nail and trim it straight across.

CALLUSES AND CORNS

Our poor feet—as we age they go from darling baby toes to veterans of the pavement wars. Calluses and corns are their battle scars. Calluses are hard pads of thickened skin that appear on the sides and soles of feet; they are caused by friction or pressure. Small hard patches on the toes with a plug of skin at the center are called corns.

Smoothing Skin: Calluses can be removed with a pumice stone after soaking them for five minutes in a solution of dish liquid and apple cider vinegar. Corns will likewise vanish if you massage in castor oil or a capsule of vitamin A or E and cover them with a cotton sock. For a really old-time remedy, soak an onion slice in white vinegar and bandage it over the corn overnight.

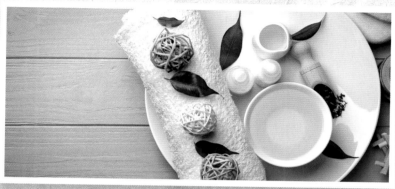

Spa composition with tea tree oil

DIABETIC FOOT CARE

For people with type-2 diabetes, maintaining foot health is critical. Foot wounds, ingrown toenails, and blisters that break the skin may heal slowly, leading to circulatory complications, ulcers, and possible amputation. Roughly 15 percent of diabetics will develop these ulcers. The loss of sensation in the extremeties, called neuropathy, can also hide small punctures or cuts. See your doctor if you find any foot wounds.

Speed Is Essential: Never wait to tend a diabetic's foot wounds. Treat open cuts or sores with ozonated olive oil—which delivers oxygen to the affected area, helping it to heal faster—and with aloe gel. Natural salves, such as goldenseal, are also safe because they have no side effects.

DIY: Curing Athlete's Foot

The fungus that causes this contagious condition—with its itching and burning between the toes, peeling skin, blisters, discolored nails, and scaly patches—is called *Trichophyton mentagrophytes*, and it is found anywhere that is warm and moist. To treat it, place 40 drops of tea tree oil in a basin of water and soak your feet for 10 minutes. Dab neem oil between your toes with a cotton ball, or make a strong oregano tea and use it as a soak twice daily. For a traditional remedy, place slices of fungicidal garlic between the toes—or take garlic supplements.

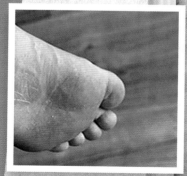

Athlete's foot

JOINT PROBLEMS

Joints are the junctions where bones—and their supporting structures—meet, and as such they are vulnerable to overextending and twisting injuries. A number of natural remedies have a long tradition of treating joint problems.

Human joints are found in the neck, shoulders, elbows, wrists, fingers, spine, hips, knees, ankles, and toes, and are held in place by a network of muscles, tendons, ligaments, and cartilage. They range from the immovable joints located in the skull to the flexible ball-and-socket architecture of the hip.

Any joints that move are prone to damage from sports, falls, horseplay, or auto accidents. Injuries include strains, the twisting or stretching of the tendons that connect to bones, and which often occur from repeated motions; sprains, the sudden, acute tearing or stretching of ligaments around a joint; tendonitis, a painful inflammation of the tendons; and bursitis, an inflammation of the fluid-filled sacs that lubricate a joint. Beside icing, heat, and Epsom salt baths, there are herbal treatments that can ease pain and tenderness and restore mobility.

HEALTHY SOLUTIONS
The following herbal remedies can help you decrease swelling and ease the pain of strains, sprains, tendon inflammation, and bursitis.

Olive Oil: Massage the oil into the affected area for 10 minutes twice a day. It has both pain-relieving and anti-inflammatory effects.

Olive oils

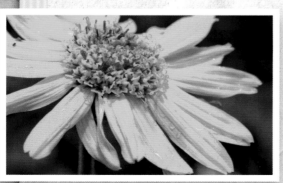

Arnica: This anti-inflammatory herb has a long tradition of treating joint discomfort as well as swelling and bruising. Apply arnica gel, cream, or ointment to any painful area where there is no broken skin.

Arnica

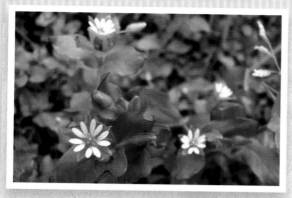
Chickweed

Chickweed: This herb has long been a valued treatment for joint problems. It is rich in nutrients such as vitamins and minerals and is also an analgesic and anti-inflammatory. Make a paste from the herb and apply it over the affected area, then wipe off with a damp cloth once it has dried. You can also drink an infusion of chickweed.

Sage: This powerful herb has a number of healing properties. Make a healing rub by crushing a handful of sage leaves in your hands and then simmering them with apple cider for 10 minutes. Soak a cloth in the mixture and apply it to the inflamed area.

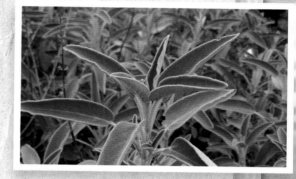
Sage

Cayenne: This hot pepper contains the pain reliever capsaicin. Add a tablespoon to a few cups of warm water and use it as a foot or hand soak or on a compress. Or prepare a muscle rub by combining 3 tablespoon cayenne with 1 cup olive oil and heating over a double boiler. Add ½ cup grated beeswax and keep stirring until melted. Chill for 10 minutes, whisk, chill another 15 minutes, then whisk again. Place rub in a covered glass jar and store in the refrigerator for up to a week.

White Willow Tea: This pain treatment dates back to the ancient Greeks. The plant's salicin converts to salicylic acid, similar to the active ingredient in aspirin. Combine 2 teaspoons of powdered or chipped white willow bark with 1 cup boiling water, steep for 30 minutes, then strain. Add honey and lemon to taste; use twice a day.

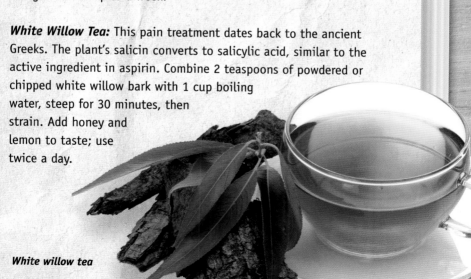
White willow tea

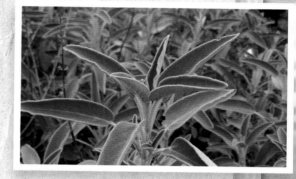

BACK PAIN

Back pain is one of the major causes of workplace absenteeism, costing the United States $100 billion in lost income and productivity. In addition to exercise, herbal treatments can ease suffering by reducing pain and swelling.

Whether back pain is caused by long hours in front of a computer, a lifting injury or fall, a gym workout gone wrong, arthritis, a bad mattress, pregnancy, or age, the condition usually reflects an injury to the muscles, ligaments, or spinal disks in the back. In addition to pain and spasms, symptoms may also include a slight fever, swelling, numbing of the buttocks, pain extending to the legs and knees, and pain that increases after sitting for long periods. It's important to address back pain before you begin losing sleep or find yourself unable to work or perform even simple physical tasks.

STEPS TO WELLNESS

Icing, heating, and gentle exercises and stretching can help mild to moderate back pain, as can warn Epsom salt baths, but there are also natural healing agents that are quite effective. For extreme back pain, make sure to see your physician.

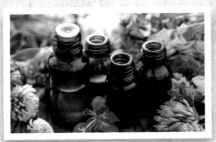

Essential oils

Essential Oils: These powerful oils have anti-inflammatory, antispasmodic, and analgesic effects on swollen, aching tissues. Try massaging one of these oils into the affected area: 3 or 4 drops of lavender oil twice daily; 5 or 6 drops of peppermint oil with 1 tablespoon of a carrier oil twice daily; 1 tablespoon warmed castor oil or olive oil once daily.

Fenugreek: Make a pain-easing tonic with a glass of hot milk, 1 teaspoon fenugreek powder, and a touch of honey. Drink every night. Fenugreek has anti-inflammatory properties and is believed to relieve pain.

Ginger: This age-old remedy requires 1 or 2 inches of fresh

Fenugreek

Ginger

ginger steeped for 5 to 10 minutes in hot water. Add honey to taste and drink twice daily.

Turmeric: This is a popular curative in India: add a teaspoon of turmeric to a glass of hot milk and drink twice daily. The compound curcumin found in this spice is both an anti-inflammatory and a pain reliever.

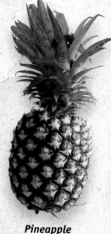

Turmeric

Basil leaves: Steep 1 or 2 tablespoons of fresh basil leaves in hot water for 10 minutes; add honey to taste, and take 2 or 3 times daily. Or you can apply basil oil directly to the affected part of your back. Basil contains anti-inflammatory and analgesic oils such as eugenol, citronellol, and linalool.

Basil

Pineapples: Blend together a half cup of fresh pineapple chunks and a cup of water or eat a half cup of pineapple; do this daily. Pineapples contain the enzyme bromelain, which, among other things, acts to reduce swelling and pain.

Pineapple

Quick Fixes: You can drink chamomile tea or ¼ to ½ cup of aloe vera juice to receive similar healing effects. A warm glass of milk also has anti-inflammatory properties. Vitamins C, D, and E can also help when treating back problems, but it's healthiest to increase your intake through fruits and vegetables rather than supplements.

DIY: The Old Garlic Cure

This is a traditional back treatment your grandmother would approve of. Smash 8 to 10 cloves of garlic into a fine paste, then apply the paste to your back. Cover the area with a towel and rest for half an hour. Then clean your back with a damp cloth. Apply twice daily. Garlic contains selenium and capsaicin, which both possess anti-inflammatory and painkilling effects.

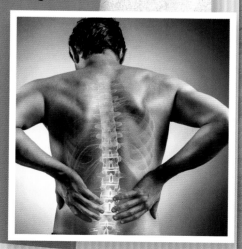

HEADACHES

Few things intrude on a person's day like the throbbing, deep-seated pain of a bad headache. Migraine sufferers often have to take to darkened bedrooms until their misery subsides. Happily, a bounty of pain-suppressing herbs and botanicals can help.

Headache pain can be sharp and squeezing, or dull and thudding; it can come and go or provide a steady throb; feel mild or intense or a mixture of both. Even though the brain itself has no fibers to feel pain, the surrounding tissue, arteries, veins, and nerves are easily inflamed. They can be triggered by fatigue, stress, allergies, eyestrain, poor posture, alcohol, drugs, hormones, or blood sugar. They may also be hereditary.

Headaches are classified into primary headaches: tension, migraine, and cluster; secondary headaches, such as sinus headaches, caused by disease, drug abuse, or structural damage to the head or neck; and cranial neuralgia, which includes facial pain.

HEAD BANGERS

Tension headaches are perhaps the most common, although researchers are still not sure what causes them. It may be contractions of the muscles that cover the skull, possibly caused by strenuous labor, sitting at a computer and focusing for any length of time, or high levels of stress or anxiety. They are characterized by mild or moderate pain on both sides of the head. Cluster headaches appear at the same time each day for a week or so, and then go away for months or years. They may be triggered by changes in sleep habits or certain medications, resulting in a sudden flooding of histamines and serotonin in the brain. The pain is described as excruciating and is usually located behind one eye. Inflamed sinuses cause pressure and pain that emanate from your forehead, cheeks, and the bridge of your nose.

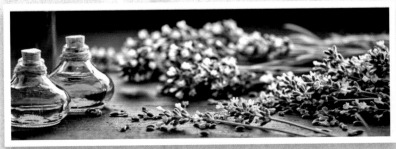

Oils

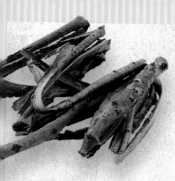

Willow bark

Pain Management: It is possible to relieve headache pain without resorting to over-the-counter medications, although one painkilling remedy, willow bark, contains a compound that is a close cousin to aspirin. Taking magnesium is also very effective; many migraine sufferers have low levels of the mineral. Taking 200 to 600 mg daily can reduce the frequency of attacks. Peppermint or lavender oil applied to the forehead provide a cooling sensation and bring blood flow to the area as well as reduce muscle contractions. If necessary, dilute the essential oils with almond, grapeseed, or coconut oil. Applying a topical preparation of cayenne pepper can relieve headache pain, reduce inflammation, and relax muscles. Capsaicin, a compound found in the pepper, depletes the element that creates pain, called substance P.

MIGRAINE HEADACHES

The intensity and duration of these headaches can lay sufferers low for more than a day. Symptoms may include pain, visual auras, nausea, vomiting, and sensitivity to light and noise.

Herbal Relief: Based on a recent study, inhaling lavender oil for 15 minutes can reduce the intensity of migraines. Out of 129 reported attacks, 92 reponded to the herb. Feverfew supplements are known to prevent the onset of migraines, reduce their frequency, and treat their symptoms. Try a dose of 50 to 100 mg. Butterbur is an herb that reduces the inflammatory effect of chemicals that bring on headaches, especially migraines. A dose of 75 mg twice a day is recommended.

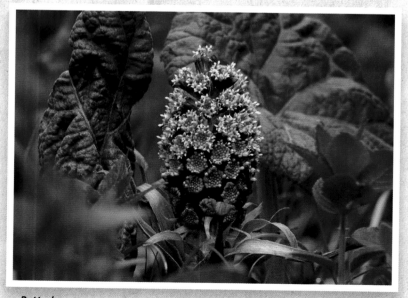

Butterbur

DENTAL HEALTH

People are typically judged on their appearance and one of the first things that others notice is an even, white smile—or the lack of one. Poor dentition also has serious health implications, so pay attention to proper dental care.

The human mouth is a repository for an astonishing amount of bacteria—one tooth might be host to more than five million. It's no

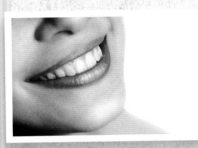

An attractive smile is an asset

wonder that even a small wound to the gums is soon swollen and sore. When you add viruses and fungi to the mix, you end up with bad breath, decaying teeth, canker sores, cold sores, thrush, abscesses, and gum disease. Regular visits to a dentist are critical for keeping the mouth healthy, especially as people age and their teeth begin to loosen or shift.

The loss of even one tooth can have serious implications for the whole mouth.

AT-HOME TOOTH CARE

Brushing twice a day is hammered into us since childhood. It still stands. If you miss the late shift, all those bacteria remain in your mouth overnight. In addition to brushing with a soft brush, you should gently floss between your teeth or use a water pik, and then rinse with an antiseptic mouthwash. A tongue scraper

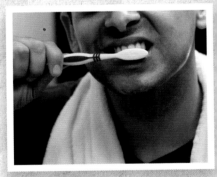

Brush regularly

removes even more bacteria to combat bad breath.

Herbal Mouthwash: Cloves make a refreshing antibacterial mouthwash. Combine a cup of boiling water with 1 tablespoon of whole cloves in a glass canning jar, then strain when cooled. Use one teaspoon as a gargle twice a day. It will keep for up to a week. Cold rosemary tea also makes an antibacterial gargle.

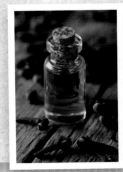

CAVITIES

Tooth decay most often occurs when carbohydrates left on the teeth mix with bacteria, acids, and saliva, and form a sticky substance called plaque that eats into tooth enamel. The results are damaged, unstable teeth and pain when the decay enters the tender pulp. Although children are more cavity prone than adults, decay can occur at any time, especially if a tooth is cracked or if fillings are loose.

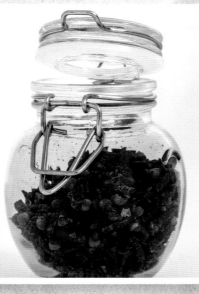

Cloves

Keep Decay Away: Reducing sugar and sweets is one way to keep teeth sound. Chose a diet rich in nutrients and fat-soluble vitamins such as A, D, E, and K, and one low in processed foods. Take echinacea, goldenseal, plaintain, and propolis to prevent decay and help strengthen teeth. For toothache pain, gargle with cayenne in warm water and apply oil of cloves.

GUM DISEASE

Another cause of mouth pain is gum disease, an infection of the tissues caused by plaque; symptoms include bleeding or swollen gums, loose teeth, and bad breath. It can be caused by poor hygiene, lack of flossing, smoking, medications, and pregnancy.

Ease Your Gums: Oil of cloves is the go-to here—massage the oil directly into your gums for pain relief; or use two drops of tea tree or nutmeg oil in a carrier oil. Increase your intake of vitamin C, and add crushed garlic to salads and hot dishes.

Quick tips: For the occasional canker sore on your gums, swish chamomile or sage tea inside you mouth or eat fermented foods to restore beneficial mouth fauna. If you are prone to cold sores, soothe them with aloe vera gel or make a lemon balm tea compress; take a lysine supplement to prevent outbreaks.

WHO'S WHO?

There are a number of medical professionals who work on the teeth and mouth, and it helps to know what tasks each one performs. Dentists take care of the teeth and superficial gum issues; dental hygienists clean the teeth; endodontists work on the interiors of teeth, which includes root canal treatment; periodontists specialize in gum disease; and oral surgeons treat the hard and soft tissue of the mouth, face, and jaw, including the removal of teeth.

SKIN AILMENTS

Among the conditions that target the skin are disfiguring diseases, inflammation, burns, rashes, and bacterial, viral, and fungal invaders. Neglecting skin problems can have systemic—and cosmetic—consequences, so speedy treatment is essential.

Human skin is composed of three layers: the waterproof epidermis, which protects it from pathogens and water loss; the dermis, home to connective tissue, hair follicles, and sweat glands; and the hypodermis, a layer of fat and connective tissue that contains large blood vessels and nerves. There are nine conditions that affect the skin: rashes; bacterial infections; viral infections; fungal infections; parasitic infections; pigmentation disorders; tumors; trauma, including wounds and burns; and an uncategorized group that includes wrinkles, rosacea, and varicose veins.

BACTERIAL INFECTIONS

When certain bacteria penetrate the skin through a wound, they will multiply and attack the underlying tissues. The body responds by sending white blood cells to battle the invaders by producing antibodies that target certain pathogens. A bacterial skin infection is usually accompanied by pain, swelling, redness, and warmth.

Trusted Healers: Many herbal remedies have become indispensable for wound care. Yarrow stops bleeding, speeds healing, and fights infection. Apply as a poultice directly on the wound. Calendula petals can be used in tinctures to wash wounds and ointments to treat infections and increase circulation. Comfrey reduces the

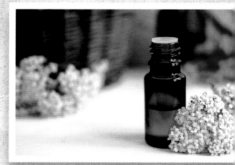

Yarrow oil

inflammation of bruises, but should not be used on open wounds. Tea tree oil applied topically can prevent infection and aid healing. Plantain is excellent at fighting infection and soothing skin. Aloe can also cool and soothe inflamed skin. Moistened chamomile tea bags make great compresses to reduce swelling and redness.

VIRAL INFECTIONS

Viral skin infections include varicella, the childhood disease known as chicken pox; herpes zoster, or shingles, a debilitating rash caused by a reactivation of the chicken pox virus; herpes simplex, which includes cold sores and genital herpes; and molluscum contagiosum, which causes pearl-like bumps on the skin.

Virus-Fighting Herbs: Viral infections do not respond to antibiotics. Antiviral herbs focus on increasing immunity, allowing the body's own defense system to attack the pathogens, as opposed to antiviral drugs that target only specific pathogens. Elderberries are renowned flu fighters, combating both A and B strains. Echinacea is known for boosting the immune system. Calendula contains high levels of flavonoids that protect cells from free radicals and attack viruses. Garlic has antiviral compounds, as do astragalus root, cat's claw, ginger, licorice root, and elderberry.

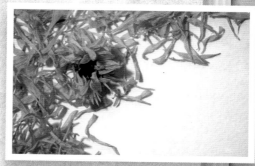
Calendula petals

RASHES

Rashes are areas of inflamed or itchy red skin or raised spots caused by allergies, irritation, infection, disease, or blocked pores. Examples include acne, dermatitis, eczema, hives, and psoriasis.

Skin Soothers: Treat eruptions with aloe vera, witch hazel, or apple cider vinegar; apply a warm chamomile or black tea compress to itchy outbreaks; press on fresh basil leaves or peppermint leaves, or make a turmeric poultice to reduce inflammation. Use red clover to calm eczema flare-ups. Treat acne with tea tree oil, sweet basil tea, olive oil, and hemp, safflower, or rose hip oil.

ADDITIONAL REMEDIES

Fungal Infections: For problems such as athlete's foot, applications of garlic, black walnut, tea tree oil, calendula, licorice, chamomile, and oregano may be effective.

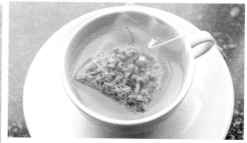
Chamomile tea

Burns: For superficial burns, use applications of aloe, plantain, and slippery elm; prepare a calendula or lavender oil cold compress; or create a comfrey salve with coconut oil. Echinacea will heal burns and acne.

BITES, STINGS, AND POISON PLANTS

It really can be a jungle out there, especially during the times of year—notably spring and summer—when biting, stinging insects and toxic plants abound. Keep your eyes open and keep a supply of natural remedies at the ready.

No matter what part of the country you live in, there is definitely some insect menace that is going to set its sights on you and come calling—and leave you with a red, swollen, itchy memento. Even in the busiest city, you will encounter the stray mosquito or bumblebee. Country and suburban homes alike are beset by mosquitoes, black flies, deer flies, ticks, deer ticks, spiders, bees, wasps, and hornets. In addition, Southerners have biting fire ants.

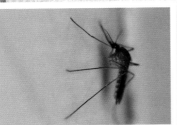

Mosquito

DON'T BUG OUT

You can keep mosquitoes and most flying insects away by applying oil of citronella, lemon balm, catnip, marigold, basil, and lavender to the skin.

Ease the Itch: Treat itchy mosquito bites with an application of aloe gel, apple cider vinegar, baking soda paste, raw honey, or a hot compress of black tea.

Soothe the Sting: When honeybees sting, they inject venom and leave their stingers embedded in the skin. First remove the stinger by flicking the edge of a playing card over it, then wash the wound with mild soap. Neutralize

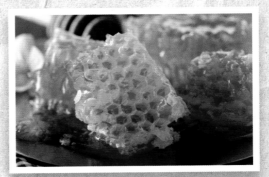

Natural honey

the venom of bee, wasp, and hornet stings with lavender essential oil, baking soda or Epsom salt paste, toothpaste, meat tenderizer (the enzyme papain breaks down toxins), honey, or crushed basil leaves. Use ice to reduce swelling. Anyone with an anaphylactic reaction to insect stings needs to carry an EpiPen.

Repel Icky Ticks and Invasive Fleas: Ticks carry diseases—most notable is Lyme disease, carried by deer ticks—that they transmit when they bite into their hosts and engorge themselves with blood. Fleas often come inside on humans or pets, and begin feeding. Keep both biting nuisances away by using lavender, garlic, pennyroyal, pyrethrum (chrysanthemum), sage, and eucalyptus.

Spider Woes: Gardeners sometimes get swollen spider bites on the face and hands, but most are harmless. (It helps to learn to identify the poisonous spiders in your region.) Clean a minor bite with mild soap. Draw out toxins with baking soda, aspirin, or activated charcoal paste, or prepare a grated raw potato poultice.

POISONOUS PLANTS

If you enjoy gardening or hiking, it helps if you can recognize toxic plants such as poison ivy, poison oak, and sumac. Otherwise you are at risk for a nasty, lingering rash. Every part of these plants contains urushiol, an oil that causes an allergic reaction, or histamine response, in most of the population. This rash is characterized by red, swollen skin, weepy blisters, and severe itching. Although the rash will clear up in one to three weeks, the oil lingers on tools and clothing indefinitely. Gardeners who fear exposure to poison plants should always wear cloth gloves—the urushiol can penetrate latex.

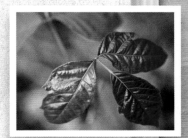

Poison ivy

Triple Threat: Poison ivy (*Toxicodendron radicans*) has pointy leaves arranged in threes that turn red in fall. Poison oak leaves (*T. diversilobum*) are a cross between oak leaves and poison ivy. Look for greenish-yellow or white berries; the plant is on the West Coast only. Poison Sumac (*T. vernix*) is a woody shrub found in the Southeast, with odd-numbered leaflets in pairs and glossy, pale yellow berries.

Treat the Rash: Wash with strong soap if there is exposure to toxic

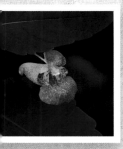

plants. If a rash appears, apply compresses of black tea—its tannins reduce inflammation—apple cider vinegar, or witch hazel. Ease intense itching with a compress with a few drops of jewelweed, geranium, rose, or lavender oil. Bentonite clay and colloidal oatmeal baths are also effective. A compress of one part echinacea tincture to three parts water can lower histamine reactions.

Jewelweed

HAIR AND NAIL CARE

You can use conditioners and oil treatments to beautify your hair and nails, but the true secret to healthy keratin is what happens on the inside. Herbs and supplements, used inside and out, will help you look polished from your head to your fingertips.

Sleek, glossy hair and smooth, unblemished nails are not only indicators of good health, they also promote self-confidence. But so often hair and nails are lackluster, dry, and damaged. This can be due to poor diet, coloring/polishing, overstyling, stress, hormonal changes, aging, and medications. Increasing your intake of keratin-benefiting supplements and herbs is a good first step to encourage new growth; follow this by creating

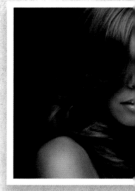

Lustrous hair

herbal remedies to treat the hair, scalp, nails, and cuticles. You can take biotin supplements or prepare an overnight biotin scalp massage by crushing 3 tablets and combining them with olive oil. Vitamins E and C are also effective for hair and nail growth, both taken internally or massaged onto the scalp in a carrier oil.

CROWNING GLORY

Always treat your hair delicately—no hard pulling when dry or wet and no overbraiding or overdrying—and be sure to nourish it from within.

Oil Massage: In addition to olive oil, try using coconut, rosemary, castor, almond, argan, jojoba, and vitamin E oils as scalp rubs. They can be left on for a few hours or overnight under a shower cap.

Essential Oils: These antioxidant-rich oils that cleanse pores and promote new hair growth need to be added to a few tablespoons of a carrier oil such as olive, almond, or coconut. They include evening primrose, flaxseed, saw palmetto, sage, lavender, peppermint, tea tree, black seed, neem, pumpkin seed, eucalyptus, and lemongrass.

Aloe Vera: Twice a week, cut open an aloe vera leaf and apply the gel to your scalp. Wait an hour and then rinse with a gentle shampoo. The proteolytic enzymes in aloe clear dead cells from the scalp and stimulate hair follicles.

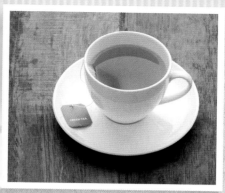

Green tea

Green Tea: Soak a green tea bag in hot water for 8 minutes, then press the tea all over your scalp. Leave on for an hour, then rinse with cool water. Other growth-boosting teas include bamboo, nettle, sage, and black tea.

Cayenne: Mix 1 teaspoon cayenne pepper with 2 teaspoons olive oil and apply to your hair, especially areas where it might be thinning. Leave on for 10 minutes, then rinse with cool water. Perform twice a month.

Mustard seed: To encourage hair growth and minimize loss, massage a tablespoon of mustard seed oil into your scalp, cover hair with plastic wrap, and wait for 30 minutes. Then shampoo as usual. Repeat once a week.

Mustard seed oil

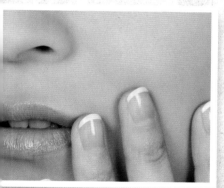

Healthy nails

ATTRACTIVE NAILS

Whether you're a woman or a man, achieving clean, healthy nails should be part of your basic grooming process. Still, our nails can take a beating from everyday tasks, so be sure to pamper them at least once a week.

Cuticle Balm: This emollient mixture of aromatic oils will soften and heal damaged cuticles. Combine 1 tablespoon jojoba oil and 1 tablespoon avocado oil with 10 drops tea tree oil and 10 drops lavender oil in a dark glass jar and shake well. Massage a few drops into the cuticles of the fingers and toes every few days.

Nettle Tea: This ancient treatment for stronger, longer nails provides vital nutrients the body requires to produce nail tissue. Add 3 teaspoons of dried nettle to a cup of hot water and steep for 10 minutes. Add honey or blackstrap molasses (another nail builder) to taste.

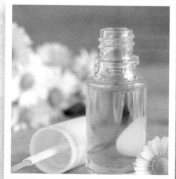

Cuticle care

COMBATING WEIGHT ISSUES

Many people find that as they age, they begin to carry more weight. But statistics indicate that today even children and teens in the United States are at an increased risk for obesity due to high-fat diets and poor exercise habits.

Everyone knows that extra weight, over time, can be harmful to the heart, lungs, circulation, joints, and organs. But dieting is hard. Unlike harmful habits such as smoking, that can be stopped cold, dieters still need to consume food every day; plus food is not intrinsically harmful, so moderation remains the key when trying to lose weight.

BUMP UP METABOLISM

Weight loss is not just about reducing your foot intake or focusing on healthier choices. You need to increase your metabolism and rate of digestion so that you burn more calories—and shed more fat. Exercise is one way to do this, but there are also many herbal options. The herbs and spices listed below are especially effective if you have hit that proverbial wall and are not losing any weight while continuing to stick to your diet.

Ginseng: This powerful metabolism booster can keep your energy levels high. Take 15–20 drops of ginseng extract in tea or water twice a day, or take 5 grams of ginseng extract twice a day for 2 weeks, then reduce to 2 grams.

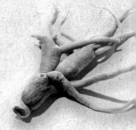

Ginseng

Hibiscus: This vivid red tea helps to rid the body of excess water. It also has an enzyme called phaseolamin, which can inhibit the production of amylase, the enzyme that turns carbs into sugar molecules, thus limiting the amount of carbs the body absorbs. It is low in calories and, like most teas, it takes the edge off your appetite.

Recipe: Combine 2 teaspoons dried hibiscus flowers with two cups boiling water in a teapot, then let steep for 5 minutes. Strain and add honey to taste.

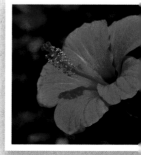

Hibiscus

Yerba mate: This traditional South American beverage is made from the aged and dried yerba mate plant. Its phytonutrients elevate energy levels, suppress appetite, boost mood, and aid in weight loss by inhibiting the enzymes that metabolize fat and slowing the emptying of the stomach.

Recipe: Add 1 tablespoon dried yerba mate to a teapot, add two cups hot (not boiling) water, and let it steep for 5 minutes. Strain and sip.

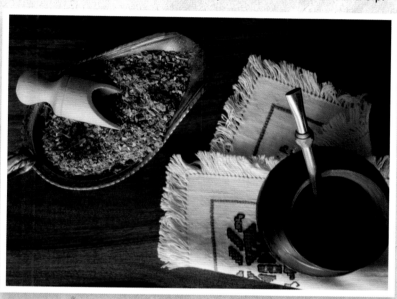

Yerba mate

Goji berries: These tasty fruits make an ideal snack—a quarter cup serving combined with nuts is crunchy and satisfying. Sprinkle them over yogurt, salads, or breakfast cereals, or add them to a fruit smoothie.

Quick fixes: Hot herbal teas are filling, low calorie, and nutrient rich. Make cinnamon tea by boiling 1 cup of water and adding 1 teaspoon plus a cinnamon stick. Or combine 1 teaspoon green tea and ½ teaspoon ground ginger, 1 teaspoon each dried dandelion leaves and peppermint, or 2 teaspoons dried sage or a handful of chopped sage for a stress-busting beverage. Mix ¼ teaspoon black pepper in warm water with honey to taste, or you can make a cold drink by adding ¼ teaspoon cayenne pepper and the juice of half a lime to a cup of water.

THE AYURVEDIC WAY

Traditional Indian medicine offers a number of less-familiar but effective weight-loss aids. These include a gum resin called guggal that stimulates thyroid function; pu-erh, a fermented Chinese tea that aids digestion; coleus forskohlii root, a thyroid stimulant that increases energy; and gurmar leaf, an Indian vine that is used to treat obesity and diabetes. For sourcing information, check the internet.

COPING WITH INSOMNIA

As the world around us speeds up and stressors at home and work increase, sleep may begin to elude us. Insomnia, the inability to find restful sleep, is an ancient malady but one with many natural treatments.

It is estimated that millions of people worldwide suffer from insomnia—the inability to fall asleep in a timely manner or to remain asleep without repeatedly awakening. Some 30 to 40 percent of Americans experience it each year. Sleep is necessary for humans to function. It is a key factor in maintaining metabolism and immunity, as well as memory and learning: during sleep is when the daily information received by the brain is collected into the long-term memory.

UP ALL NIGHT

Many people who are plagued with insomnia say they are unable to "turn off" their brains at night, that there is too much input or noise. The concerns of the day, plus long-term worries, seem to concentrate in the mind at bedtime.

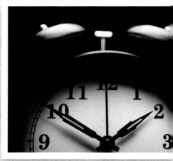

Even ticking clocks can disrupt sleep

In addition to a buildup of stress, insomnia can be caused by medical or psychiatric conditions, medications, disruption of circadian rhythms, poor sleep habits, lifestyle choices, biological factors, pregnancy, and hormone levels. There is even evidence that exposure to the light from electronic devices just before bedtime is a culprit. Over time, sleep deprivation can cause daytime fatigue, fogginess, depression, and lack of concentration.

Relaxation Practices: Whatever the cause, there are a number of ways to relax the body and ease the mind into sleep. Try a yoga position called savasana, or corpse pose, where you lay on your back with your arms at your sides, legs slightly apart. Beginning with your toes, clench the muscles for 5 seconds, then relax them for 30 seconds. Repeat this process up the entire length of your body. Or try meditating: focus your mind on a single, internal image, letting thoughts wander into your head without reacting to them. You can take a melatonin supplement—melatonin is a hormone that regulates sleep—or drink a glass of milk before bed; milk contains tryptophan, an amino acid in the brain that causes sleepiness. Micronutrients such as the B vitamins, iron, copper, and magnesium can also help to regulate sleep patterns.

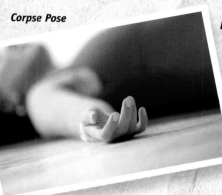

Corpse Pose

Natural Slumber: Insomnia has been impacting humans for thousands of years, so there are numerous time-tested herbal solutions. These herbs are a far safer option for inducing sleep than medications that can be addictive or cause episodes of sleepwalking. Valerian root is a reliable sleep aid; if your body builds up a tolerance for it, switch to another herbal remedy for a few weeks, then go back to valerian. Passionflower extract contains the neurotransmitter GABA, which relaxes muscles and nerves. California poppy is an effective sedative that eases restlessness and can even be given to children. South American mulungu tree bark (*Erythrina mulungu*) combats both anxiety and insomnia,

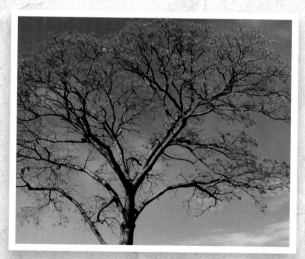

Mulungu tree

while hops are an effective sedative that can increase sleep time. For infrequent bouts of insomnia, try the calming effects of lavender or chamomile tea just before bedtime.

Return to Sleep: For those who suffer morning insomnia—awakening before it's time to get up, possibly due to a spike in cortisol levels—there are specific herbs to address the problem. Ashwagandha is an ayurvedic herb that reduces stress, anxiety, and cortisol levels, and allows a return to sleep. Magnolia bark, a part of Chinese medicine, can reduce cortisol levels and promote relaxation.

IMPROVING MEMORY

Whether you've always been a little absentminded or find yourself becoming more forgetful as you age, there are a number of herbs and botanicals that can both sharpen the brain and restore a faulty memory.

The brain, like the heart, keeps working around the clock. Some researchers believe it uses sleep time to renew itself, like a cell phone plugged into a dock, and it certainly uses those nightly hours to consolidate memories. Yet as we grow older, brain function begins to decrease; we experience memory loss, cognitive impairment, and fuzzy thinking. The hippocampus, the part of the brain where information is stored, begins to deteriorate. The proteins and hormones that protect brain cells start to diminish. The best aids for retaining memory include avoiding smoking and alcohol, staying active and engaged, exercising the brain with word games and puzzles, and learning new things. Another aid is using natural remedies to stay sharp and on top of things.

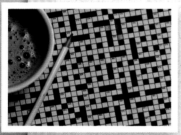
Crossword puzzle

HERBAL TONICS

Over time, natural healers recognized that certain herbs and botanicals were able to increase focus, sharpen mental skills, and enhance memory, even into old age. Many of these remedies have held up under lab scrutiny of their healing properties and some may even become valuable allies in the fight against Alzheimer's disease.

Ginkgo Biloba: This is perhaps the best-known herbal memory booster and possibly one of the oldest. It may also help to heal and regenerate brain cells and even enhance intelligence. Do not take with any blood thinners.

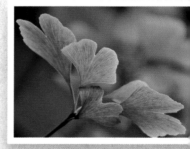
Ginkgo Biloba

Gotu Kola: This herb (*Centella asiatica*), a native of Southeast Asia, Australia, and India, is taken as a brain tonic. It not only improves blood circulation, it also supports memory function. As an adaptogen, it allows people to adapt more successfully to stressors, which can be a factor in mental fuzziness.

Ginseng: This well-regarded herb increases vitality and improves mental function. It is also an adaptogen that enables the mind and body to cope with stress; further, it may protect against the toxins that can precipitate age-related mental decline.

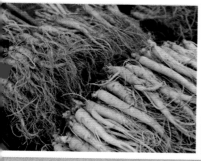

Ginseng

Vacha: Also called sweet flag (*Acorus calamus*), this is a traditional ayurvedic remedy for anxiety and other nervous disorders. It is believed to support clear thinking and aid mental focus and concentration. Its mild stimulating effect can help relieve fatigue or depression.

Rosemary: When inhaled as an essential oil in aromatherapy, this pungent kitchen favorite becomes a powerful brain booster. It can increase mental efficiency and skill and may also aid in memory retention.

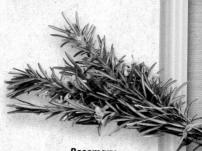

Rosemary

Bacopa: This perennial garden flower (*Bacopa monnieri*) is also an ayurvedic remedy that supports brain function as it enhances memory, heightens learning skills, and eases stress. Research indicates that it may be effective in protecting against Alzheimer's disease by reducing beta-amyloid in the brain and relieving inflammation.

Rhodiola: The root of this flowering plant (*Rhodiola rosea*) has been employed by natural healers for many years and is especially known for helping to improve brain and physical function during times of high stress. It may also alleviate anxiety, depression, and mental fatigue and aid in memory retention.

Huperzine-A: A derivative of a type of Chinese moss, this herb bolsters the brain and enhances memory. It is currently being considered as a possible preventative for Alzheimer's. It may block a certain enzyme in the brain that destroys the acetylcholine that relays information between brain cells.

Other Options: Blueberries are full of flavonoids that help to improve brain function. Green tea is loaded with antioxidants that shield proteins and lipids from age-related problems due to oxidation and also protect the hippocampus from the effects of aging. Holy basil, or tulsi, is an Indian plant (*Ocimum tenuiflorum*) that increases circulation, which oxygenates the brain, thus benefiting cognitive function.

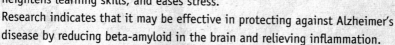

EASING DEPRESSION AND ANXIETY

Occasionally feeling emotionally out of sorts, edgy, or blue is normal for most people. If these feelings linger for weeks, however, or deepen into fear or despair, there is a risk for more serious psychological complications such as anxiety disorders and depression.

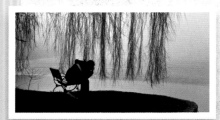

Depression often goes untreated

Every year, mental health complaints cost employers ten of billions of dollars in lost productivity in the United States. This isn't surprising, since one in five adults experiences some type of mental disorder annually. Some people seek help through counseling or therapy, some augment their sessions with medication. Antidepressants and antianxiety drugs have been a boon to many sufferers, but there is also a primary line of defense, natural remedies, that do not have the many side effects or addictive tendencies of these prescription medications.

OVERCOMING ANXIETY DISORDERS

There was once a time when anxiety was a lifesaver, when primitive humans needed lightning-fast responses to approaching danger. Today, anxiety disorders can be crippling, engendering fear and dread and bringing on panic attacks, palpitations, phobias, and paranoia that are extreme enough, in some cases, to keep the sufferer housebound. Anxiety is not a new ailment, so there is a range of effective natural treatments, or calmatives, that have been relied upon for thousands of years. Just remember not to take them in combination with prescription sedatives.

Ashwagandha: From ayurvedic medicine comes this adaptogenic herb, which eases the symptoms of anxiety and stabilizes the body's reaction to stress.

Valerian: This herbal root is quite effective against anxiety, depression, and insomnia, comparable to the prescription sedative benzodiazepine.

Valerian

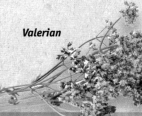

Passionflower: This herb goes back to the Aztecs as a treatment for nervous disorders; today it is recommended to relieve anxiety, stress, and insomnia. It contains GABA, an amino acid that eases tension and is effective as a muscle relaxer.

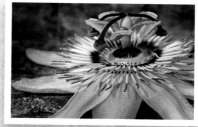

Passionflower

Lavender: Place three drops of this soothing essential oil into your palm and rub it onto your neck; or try a few drops of Roman chamomile oil to help you de-stress and calm your nerves.

WRESTLING WITH DEPRESSION

People suffering from this malady are often told to "snap out of it." But there is no easy "snap." Depression removes the normal human desire to engage and replaces it with debilitating negative thoughts. Causes include genetic predisposition, medications, personality, or an abusive environment. There may be an imbalance or lack of mood-elevating chemicals called endorphins—serotonin, dopamine, and epinephrine. Although therapists and antidepressant medications can be a lifeline to sufferers, there are also natural alternatives to consider.

Green Tea: Make this your new morning beverage. It offers the boost of caffeine, but it also contains L-theanine, which works synergistically with caffeine to elevate your mood, minus the crashing effect afterward. It also increases dopamine levels, which can help lower stress.

Chamomile Tea: This is the ideal herbal tea for later in the day. Emotional distress can often cause insomnia, and *Green tea* chamomile contains a flavonoid with relaxing properties. A cup taken in the evening with a bit of milk and honey should result in easy slumber.

Saint-John's-Wort: Since the days of ancient Greece, this herb has been used to treat emotional disorders. It contains a substance called hypericin that appears to affect the brain's neurotransmitters similar to serotonin reuptake inhibitors (SSRIs) such as Prozac or Paxil, which elevate serotonin levels.

Other Aids: Magnesium increases energy, synthesizes RNA and DNA, and stabilizes brain chemistry. The B vitamins, especially B-12 and B-6, combat stress and produce endorphins in the brain.

Note: Some herbs may interact with medications, so always check with your doctor before taking any natural remedies.

COPING WITH PREGNANCY

Even women basking in the glow of pregnancy will inevitably have to face some health side effects—many of which can be alleviated by safe herbal remedies that, furthermore, bear the stamp of approval from their female ancestors.

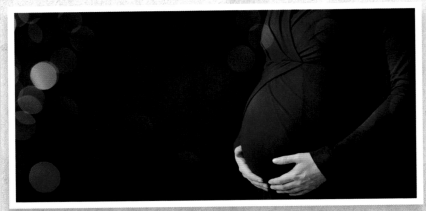

Many pregnant women swear by herbs, but always check with a physician

Women experience different issues during each of the three trimesters of pregnancy. First-trimester problems might include fatigue, nausea and morning sickness, hormonal changes, and constipation; the second trimester can bring leg cramps, varicose veins, backaches, and heartburn. During the fifth month, there may be signs of preeclampsia—high blood pressure and protein in the urine—which needs to be treated. By the third trimester, many earlier ill effects have passed, but there could be pressure on the bladder, frequent urination, backaches, hemorrhoids, shortness of breath, edema in the lower limbs, and Braxton Hicks contractions.

Other, more lasting side effects may be stretch marks on the abdomen and melasma, the "mask of pregnancy," that causes darkened gray-brown patches on the face.

SAFE AND PROTECTED

Many anxious pregnant women are seeking low-impact, non-narcotic, nonaddictive health remedies that are unlikely to harm them or their babies; these include herbs and botanicals. Still, not all herbs have been thoroughly tested on pregnant women or their babies, so always check with a doctor before taking any herbs or supplements.

Morning Sickness: For starters, avoid fatty, greasy, salty, or strong-smelling foods. Take red raspberry to ease nausea; it is loaded with vital iron and can tone the uterus, increase milk production, and even decrease labor pains. Sliced or grated fresh ginger makes an excellent cure for morning sickness. Prepare a tea by steeping a tablespoon of ginger in hot water, and adding a bit of lemon. Peppermint leaf tea also relieves queasiness and gas. Most herbal teas help women stay hydrated after bouts of nausea.

Constipation/Bladder Issues: Treat constipation with flaxseed oil and by increasing your water intake; or try taking fenugreek, slippery elm, aloe vera juice, dandelion, and nettle. Frequent urination caused by bladder irritation can be relieved with saw palmetto extract, uva ursi in tea or capsule form, or corn silk extract or capsules.

Edema: There is usually some swelling of the feet and ankles during the final trimester. Treat it by creating a relaxing footbath. Fill a basin with warm water and add ½ cup of Epsom salts and a few drops of herbal essential oils, relaxing lavender, aromatic rose, healing rosemary, or stimulating wintergreen.

Stress: During the nine months of gestation, it's important for expectant women to avoid stress. Chamomile tea has been used for centuries to promote gentle relaxation, quell nausea, ease indigestion, and relieve insomnia. Also try lavender, rhodiola, ashwagandha, holy basil, and ginseng.

> **GET IN THE KNOW**
> Mothers-to-be should have several diagnostic tests performed at specific stages. At week 20, an ultrasound is typically performed to measure and evaluate the baby and determine its sex; between weeks 26 and 28, women should be checked for signs of gestational diabetes. Older women with "geriatric" pregnancies may want to have amniocentesis performed between weeks 15 and 20 to check for chromosomal fetal abnormalities, but there is a roughly one in 100 risk of miscarriage to consider.

Stretch Marks and Melasma: Treat stretch marks with applications of aloe vera gel mixed with vitamin E oil, almond or coconut oil, or cocoa butter. Melasma patches can be lightened by combining ginseng with the Chinese herb gotu kola. Look for lotions or creams with active herbal ingredients that are known to inhibit melanin production—burdock root, mulberry, bearberry extract, Chinese sophora root, mushroom-based kojic acid; and Indian gooseberry. Gigawhite is a lightening agent that is a mix of herbs and plants that stop skin from producing melanin.

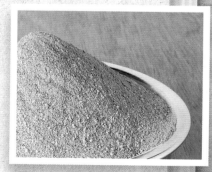

Indian gooseberry

INFANT CARE

Babies face a new, unfamiliar world and they only have one way to express their fear or discomfort: crying. So one critical requirement for herbal remedies is that they provide comfort in the face of painful colic, teething, and diaper rash.

The majority of babies are strong and remarkably resilient—they get rather squished squeezing out of a very tight spot and yet manage to look properly rounded and adorable soon after. But when things go wrong health-wise, they have no way to explain their pain or distress. New parents play a constant guessing game trying to find out what's wrong with the baby or why she won't stop crying. For anxious parents, herbal treatments can be both gentle and effective.

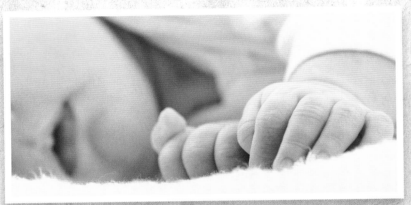

Babies often benefit from herbal calmatives

NATURAL REMEDIES

Herbs can help ease some of your baby's health problems, including the burn of diaper rash; the stress of teething, which can include pain, a slight fever, drooling, swollen gums, irritability, and refusing food; and colic. For restless babies who won't settle into sleep, herbs can take the edge off their distress without any harmful side effects—and before they reach that level of tearful frenzy that so disturbs parents.

Calming Baby: Nervines that are safe for soothing babies include chamomile, catnip, lemon balm, spearmint, rose petals, and lavender. Catnip can also be used to treat low-grade fevers, upper respiratory infections, headaches, sleep problems, and indigestion.

Colic: Make a stomach-soothing tea—that also works on teething pain—with chamomile flowers. Simply pour boiling water over 2 teaspoons of flowers, let it steep, then strain and cool. Give 1 to 2 ounces to babies, 2 to 4 ounces to children.

Diaper Rash: Make a healing "bottom wash" for the afflicted area by adding 1 cup white vinegar and ¼ teaspoon of tea tree oil to a few inches of water in a basin. Natural home remedies include applications of coconut oil, a baking-soda wash, and dry cornstarch.

Teething: Chamomile tea can be rubbed on the gums or frozen as a popsicle for baby to gnaw on. Try chamomile hydrosol, the infused water left over after the essential oil is distilled. It is much less concentrated than the oil, but has many of the same benefits. Make a soothing rub for the external jaw from 1 drop each lavender essential oil and Roman chamomile oil combined with 2 tablespoons carrier oil such as olive, almond, or coconut. Massage several drops into baby's jaw as needed. (Use only externally. Never give any essential oils to children under 2.)

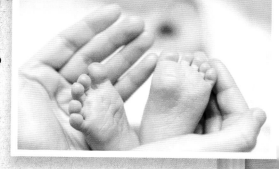

Diarrhea: In addition to feeding only bland foods—bananas, rice, applesauce—treat diarrhea with a tea made with 1 teaspoon of crushed fennel and 1 cup hot water; let it steep, then strain and cool. Give baby 2 teaspoons to sip every 2 hours. Or give 3 teaspoons of cooled antispasmodic chamomile tea. A handful of blueberries, if your child is eating solids, can also ease symptoms.

TAKE HEED

The American Academy of Pediatrics advises against giving herbs to babies under six months. Some gentle herbs that should be safe to administer are chamomile, catnip, and mint. But always check for adverse reactions when first offering anything new. Also, babies under two should never be fed honey, which can contain botulism.

Constipation: Try an herbal tea made from a peppermint tea bag or from grated ginger root. Make a healing tonic by adding equal parts licorice root and fennel seed to a pint of water; simmer for 20 minutes, then strain and cool. Give one teaspoon to baby. For babies older than 4 months, try undiluted pear or apple juice.

Fever: Catnip combined with an equal amount of dried spearmint makes an effective tea for reducing fevers. For infants, offer a teaspoon every 2 hours; for children over 3, increase it to half a cup.

SENIOR HEALTH

The golden years represent a time to savor a lifetime's accomplishments, look back at past pleasures, and plan for a proactive "third act." It's also a time when certain potentially treatable health issues should remain of concern.

Some seniors declare that "60 is the new 40," and then live up to the boast by becoming the most active, engaged, fitness-oriented, and health-conscious group of older adults in history. Their baby-boomer level of activism has turned inward, toward themselves, and they work

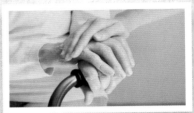
Staying active is key

hard at staying in shape and keeping up social contacts. Still, the onset of old age brings new, unfamiliar medical challenges to many senior adults—including bone-density loss, failing joints, faulty memories, and reproductive-system or sexual problems. Some of these health issues can be forestalled, or even prevented, by targeting them with specific herbs or botanicals.

PROVIDE PROPHYLAXIS

In order to maintain good health and ward off serious ailments such as cancer, heart disease, and diabetes, it makes sense to "weaponize" the immune system. The more powerful one's defenses, the less likelihood there is of facing a debilitating disease. So focus on herbs that are rich in anti-inflammatory qualities that combat pain, stiffness, swelling, and redness, and antioxidants that protect cells from free radicals.

Raise Your Defenses: Members of the *Allium* genus, including garlic and onions, are proven immunity boosters, as are American ginseng, elder flower, garlic, ginger, licorice, goldenseal, green tea, cinnamon, cayenne pepper, oregano, thyme, and turmeric.

HERBS FOR LONGEVITY

The following remedies have lengthy histories of treating the ailments and conditions that afflict older adults. Most of them are available in health-food stores and online. Always speak to your doctor before starting any herbal regimen.

Heart Health: Herbs that benefit the cardiovascular system include rosemary, turmeric, borage, nettle, ginger, valerian, ginkgo, and green tea, which can also improve pulmonary function.

Blood Sugar: Help the body regulate blood glucose levels with cinnamon, cloves, rosemary, oregano, sage, garlic, and an ayurvedic herb called *Gymnema sylvestre* or gurmar.

Arthritis: Treat the pain and swelling of joint or muscle issues with alfalfa, ginger, nettle, feverfew, cayenne pepper, turmeric, or burdock.

Osteoporosis: To strengthen bones and help prevent bone loss, try dandelion greens, nettle, safflower, and watercress.

Reproductive System Issues: Prostate problems can be addressed with Chinese ginseng, cayenne pepper, parsley, saw palmetto, or a combination of turmeric with nettle. Loss of libido may be corrected with red ginseng. Dong quai is effective for treating erectile dysfunction as well as menopause symptoms. Natural estrogens are found in anise, fennel, licorice (for seven days only), and sage.

Urinary Problems: Help restore normal kidney and bladder function with diuretics such as dandelion, nettle, and parsley and bacteria cleansers such as cranberry juice and blueberries.

Anxiety: Combat the effects of stress or nervous disorders with chamomile, lavender, valerian, ashwagandha, and passionflower.

Depression: Keep sad or negative thoughts at bay with Saint-John's-wort, valerian, lemon balm, ginger, peppermint, ginkgo, and Siberian ginseng.

Memory Loss: Help restore brain function, clear-headedness, and memory with the aid of ginkgo biloba, gotu kola, ginseng, vacha or sweet flag, rosemary, and bacopa. Huperzine-A, derived from Chinese moss, may possibly prevent Alzheimer's by facilitating information relays between brain cells.

Fatigue: Overcome frequent tiredness—or even chronic fatigue syndrome—with burdock, ginger, goldenseal, dandelion, ginkgo, valerian, licorice, milk thistle, and Saint-John's-wort.

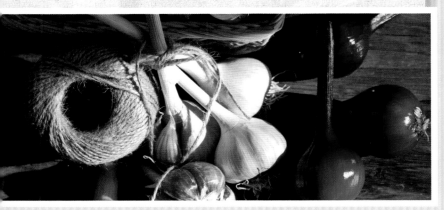

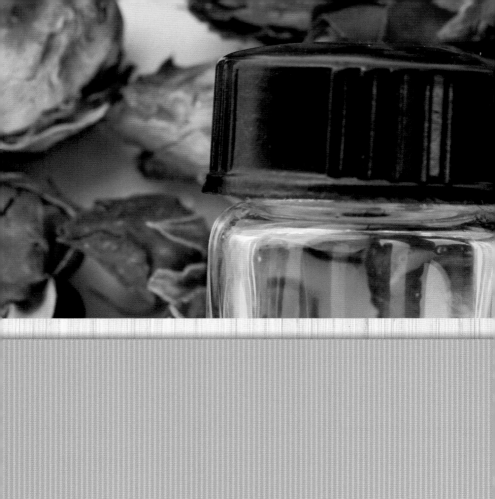
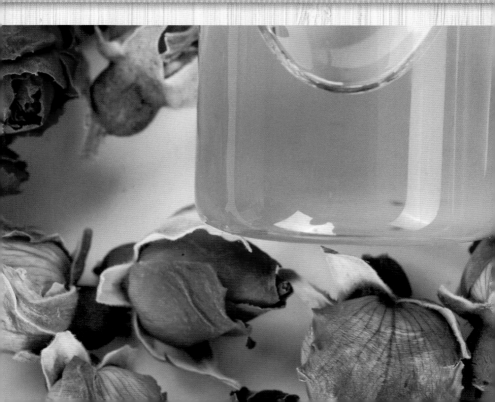

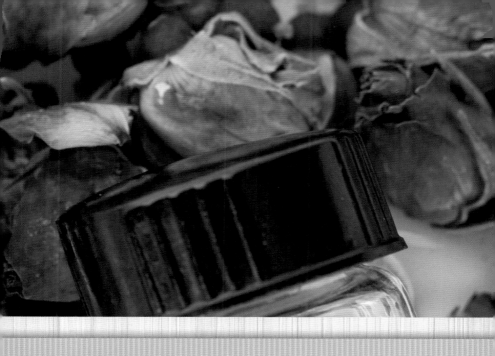

CHAPTER 4
ESSENTIAL OILS

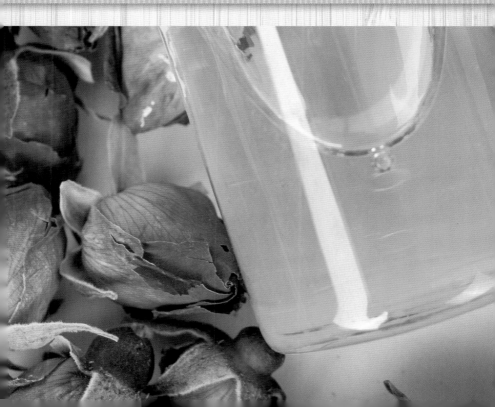

ESSENTIAL OILS

There is an almost endless list of healing possibilities offered by aromatic essential oils. Alone they maintain their character and their beneficial properties, but when blended, some can take on a wholly different "personality" than either source oil. Once used by the ancients for perfume, rituals, and embalming, today these versatile oils have been rediscovered by health enthusiasts—and are now a multibillion-dollar industry.

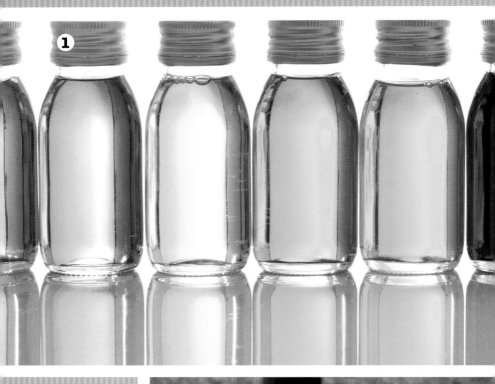

1. A variety of oils
2. Coconut oil
3. Dark bottles to protect the contents
4. Inscense stick with oils

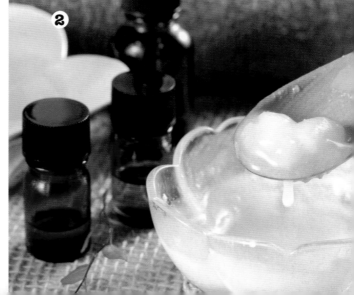

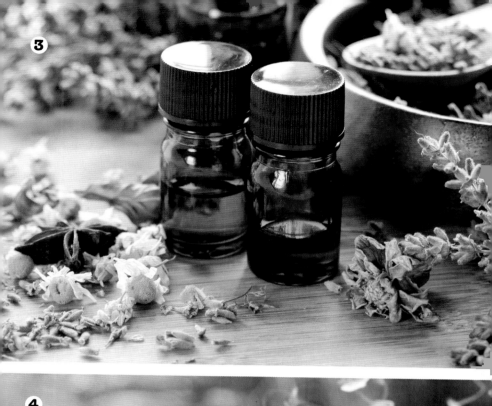

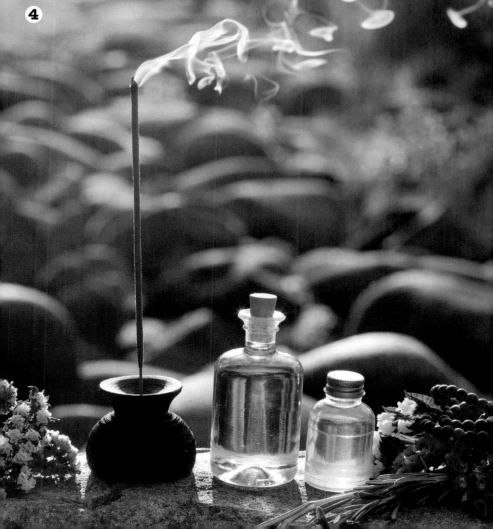

THE MODERN ADVENT OF ESSENTIAL OILS

As the natural health movement expanded in the late twentieth century, one popular "new" form of healing was the use of essential oils—concentrated oils taken from the flowers, fruits, seeds, and other parts of plants.

Technically, essential oils are hydrophobic liquids containing volatile aroma compounds from plants. The oils are essential because they capture the "essence" of a plant's fragrance (not because they are essential in terms of being indispensable). They are also ephemeral—unlike fatty oils, they evaporate without a stain when swabbed onto filter paper.

These oils date back to at least 4000 BC. Over the passing centuries, Egyptian, Greek, Roman, Persian, Chinese, and Indian cultures found a variety of uses for them:

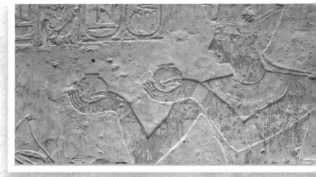

Essential oils date back to at least ancient Egypt

in aromatherapy, as topical remedies, for massage, to scent cosmetics and toiletries, and to repel pests.

In the Middle Ages, oils such as lavender, sandalwood, patchouli, and lemon were employed by healers and monks to treat sickness and disease, even the plague. Men of science kept "physic gardens," full of healing herbs and aromatic plants. But as superstitions grew and the power of the Catholic church increased, herbs and their oils fell out of use, primarily from fear of accusations of witchcraft.

During the Renaissance, herbal oils eventually came into use again, being sold openly by apothecaries, and since then their popularity with herbalists has rarely waned. But it was only relatively recently, during the rise of the counterculture in the 1960s and 1970s, that the population at large became aware of these evocative, healing oils. Patchouli oil, in particular, became a kind of "badge of inclusion" among hippies and rockers. As the new millennium approached, and the United States grew more health and fitness conscious, essential oils continued their ascent. That brings us to today, when you can't go into a health-food store without seeing a large display—if not a wall—full of essential-oil options. They are currently used in the practice of aromatherapy, as healing body scents, as perfumes, and in some cases as topical applications. They are rarely taken internally.

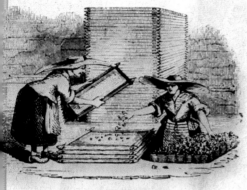

Women extracting essential oils

THE EXTRACTION PROCESS

There are many methods of extracting essential oils from plants, some going back to the early Egyptians.

Enfleurage: This ancient method involves placing flower petals on glass spread with fat; the volatile oils are transferred to the fat and then extracted using alcohol. Around the year AD 800, the Arabs developed a way to distill ethyl alcohol from sugar, thus providing a new solvent for floral essences to replace the fats that had been previously used. This knowledge spread to Europe in the Middle Ages, and certain cities, such as Grasse in France, became centers of the perfume industry.

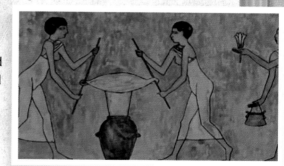

Steam Distillation: This method goes back hundreds of years and is still the most popular type of extraction. Steam is used to rupture the oil membrane of the plant and release the essential oil. The steam then travels to a condenser; as it re-liquefies, the oil floats on top, where it can be collected. The remaining water is known as hydrosol.

An early method of distilling essential oils

Expressed Oils: Citrus oils such as orange and lemon are taken from fruit rinds using a cold-press method, without heat. They are technically not essential oils, but rather therapeutic oils.

Other Methods: These include solvent extraction and the percolation method, but they do not produce therapeutic-grade essential oils.

TOP BOTANICAL SOURCES

Just as there are a number of versatile herbs that treat a range of ailments, so too are there essential oils that provide multiple medicinal benefits. Place these at the top of your "healing oils" shopping list.

THE WONDER OILS

When it comes to treating disease, illness, pain, and emotional distress, the following essential oils cover a lot of bases.

Frankincense: When used with an ultrasonic cool mist diffuser, this oil offers respiratory support for those suffering from colds, flu, bronchitis, COPD, and pneumonia. Add a drop or two to a teaspoon of carrier oil (the traditional dose for most essential oils) and massage it into the neck arteries to banish nightmares. It can balance dry or oily complexions and when applied neat to normal skin will prevent acne and blemishes. Inhaled from the bottle, it also calms and centers a brain intent upon meditation.

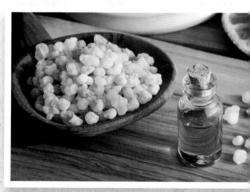

Frankincense

Clove: Well regarded as an analgesic for tooth and gum pain and for arthritis, this exotic spice is also an antifungal that can treat *Candida albicans*; an antiviral that can ease cold sores; and a natural antibacterial, useful around the house for eliminating many dangerous bacteria, including E. coli, salmonella, *H. pylori*, staphylococcus, and streptococcus. In the kitchen, add a drop to your sponge, your cutting boards, and your dish soap.

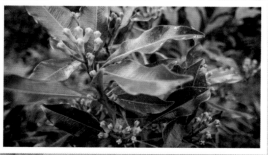

Clove bean is a common vegetable in Indonesia known for its rich nutritional values

Lavender: This bushy European herb is one of the most versatile medicinal plants; it contains more than 100 constituents including linalool, camphor, coumarins, tannins, cineole, and flavonoids. Its oil is often employed to promote calmness and sleep—dilute the oil and gently stroke it along the sides of the neck or inhale from the bottle. As a diluted topical it can ease the itch of bug bites and sunburn. It can also be mixed with aloe vera gel to soothe sun-damaged skin. In an Iranian research report from 2011, lavender was found to kill breast cancer cells, while leaving healthy cells untouched. It is often sprinkled at thresholds to repel crawling insects and, in the south of France, scorpions. Lavender is also used to flavor icings, chocolate cake, brownies, and salads.

Orange: This repository of vitamin C is also an immunity booster that can heal mouth ulcers—put a few drops of the oil in your drinking water. Don't mind the tiny sting—that means it's working. It can disinfect a wound before you bandage it and soften calluses on your feet if you rub in a few drops before donning socks and shoes. It is known to promote the production of collagen, detoxify the body, speed up circulation, and even the tone and improve the texture of skin.

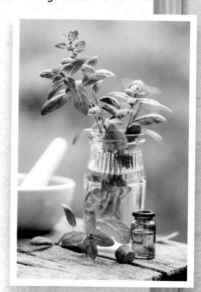

Peppermint: This aromatic oil can counteract hot flashes—place a drop on the collarbones or at the back of the neck, and the brisk cooling effect will turn down the heat. It is invaluable on a long solo road trip because it can jolt the nervous system awake and keep the brain alert. Spraying distilled water with a few drops of peppermint oil on the clothing of ADHD children just before they study has helped them concentrate. Peppermint oil is also good

Peppermint

for aching muscles; inhaling a diluted solution speeds allergy relief and loosens congestion. It is perhaps best known for calming stomach distress—take one drop in a glass of spring water for quick relief or dilute it and use it as an abdominal rub.

Oregano: This favorite of Mediterranean chefs is also a powerful microbe hunter—the oil is effective against 59 different bacterial strains. Not to mention its high levels of antioxidants allow it to combat signs of aging. Add a drop to a glass of water and gargle to soothe a sore throat. Or massage it between the toes and under the soles to ward off athlete's foot or nail fungus. Always dilute oregano oil when using it topically and avoid the eyes and mucous membranes.

TOP BOTANICAL SOURCES

Rosemary: This savory cooking herb produces an amazing essential oil—with potential to destroy several types of cancer cells based on a 2010 Turkish study. This stimulating oil also increases circulation, helping to improve varicose veins and promote clearer thinking as well as combat mental fatigue. One of the oil's phytochemicals has neuroprotective functions in brain cells, meaning it may help to prevent Alzheimer's. It can treat scalp problems such as dandruff and seborrhea by regulating oil secretion. Finally, it is known to reduce stress by lowering levels of cortisol.

Rosemary sprig

Eucalyptus: This pungent, resinous oil is a natural decongestant and expectorant—place a few drops in a bowl of hot water and lean over it with a towel draped on either side. It is a notable vasodilator that improves blood flow to the brain; this increase also aids diabetics, whose circulation is often compromised in their extremities. Biting insects stay clear of this oil, which is also able to lower a fever— place a few drops on a damp washcloth and run it over the patient's side, chest, the back of the neck, and the soles of the feet.

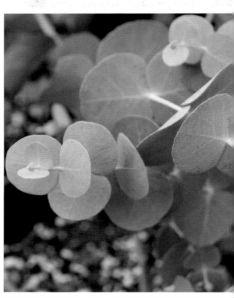

Eucalyptus plant

Tea Tree: This potent oil's anti-inflammatory properties make it very effective against skin conditions such as eczema and psoriasis. Dilute and apply several times daily. Add a few drops to your deodorant to boost its drying power. Blended with a little coconut oil, this natural antiseptic will take the heat out of razor burn after shaving. It also repels insects from both humans and pets—so use a drop or two on pet bedding or crates and apply a bit to a cotton swab to gently clean your dog's ears.

OTHER VALUED OILS

Although they may not quite be essential-oil superstars, these oils have plenty to brag about.

Basil: Both the herb and the oil are effective for treating stomach irritations, nausea, motion sickness, and flatulence; the oil acts as an appetite enhancer and increases the flow of bile. It treats respiratory infections by clearing nasal passages of mucus and harmful bacteria. In aromatherapy it treats nervous tension, mental fatigue, depression, and migraines. Basil improves metabolic functions by increasing circulation and offers relief from the pain of arthritis, burns, wounds, and sports injuries.

Basil

Juniper Berry: The essential oil's stimulating properties can treat dizziness, depression, and fatigue; it can also be used as an antiseptic on wounds. The oil can be used to detoxify the blood of harmful heavy metals, undesirable compounds, and hormones produced by the body itself.

Coriander: When inhaled, this essential oil stimulates the secretion of digestive enzymes; it also relieves colic in small children. The oil calms allergic skin reactions, such as hives, and displays antihistamine properties to help control seasonal allergies.

Coriander

Clary Sage: The essential oil's medicinal properties are antispasmodic, antidepressant, antibacterial, antiseptic, astringent, aphrodisiac, digestive, anticonvulsive, and many more. Its phytoestrogens make it one of the best herbs for balancing the body's hormones. The essential oil is also a known sleep aid, with the related benefits of easing anxiety, vertigo, and stress.

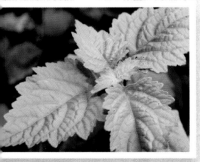

Patchouli: The steam-distilled oil possesses antidepressant, antiseptic, astringent, and aphrodisiac properties. It can be used to treat dermatitis, acne, dandruff, and eczema and to heal wounds and reduce scarring. It also offers mood- and libido-raising effects.

Patchouli

CREATE YOUR OWN BLENDS

Whether you prepare mixtures of essential oils for your own use or as gifts to give away, making them at home is easy—and a great way to provide healing or to strike a pleasing aromatic note.

In order to create your own essential-oil blends, you will need a supply of small, colored, stoppered or roller-top bottles; a plastic eye dropper; measuring cups and spoons; mixing bowls; and a starter collection of essential oils. A useful range includes lemon, orange, grapefruit, clary sage, lavender, rosemary, peppermint, eucalyptus, and tea tree. You will also need a supply of carrier oils—these dilute the strong concentrations of essential oils. Carrier oils include olive, coconut, almond, jojoba—almost any vegetable oil will do. Vodka also works.

GUIDELINES FOR BLENDING

One tip for successfully combining essential oils is picking scents that have similar attributes. For instance, stick to the floral family, the citrus family, or the woodsy family. Or blend oils that present a similar character—all calming, all stimulating, all sensual.

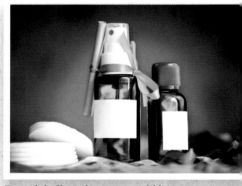

Essential oils makeup-removal kit

Basic Recipe: Add the amount of essential oil indicated in the recipe to a 10 ml bottle, then fill the rest of the bottle with your carrier oil. Below are some options for creating healing mixes and distinctive aromatic blends.

The Go-Getter: Jump-start your motivation—blend 5 drops black pepper, 5 drops lime, 5 drops orange, and 5 drops frankincense with carrier oil. Use on wrists twice daily.

The Itch Beater: Soothe irritated bug bites or inflamed rashes with 12 drops of lavender and 8 drops of peppermint in a carrier oil.

The Perk Me Up: Combine 12 drops of eucalyptus, 8 drops of rosemary, and 6 drops of grapefruit oil in a carrier for an instant energy boost. Apply to temples and wrists.

Fast Heal: Use this on superficial wounds and cuts: combine 7 drops lavender, 7 drops tea tree oil, and 7 drops frankincense oil with a carrier. Or switch out the tea tree for 5 drops peppermint for an effective headache remedy; apply to temples and back of neck.

Allergy Blend: Try this when hay fever season hits. Mix 5 drops lavender, 5 drops lemon, and 5 drops peppermint oil in a carrier. Apply under chin and to back of neck.

The Big Kahuna: This recipe creates a strong dose of healing and calming—10 drops marjoram, 10 drops frankincense, and 10 drops lemongrass oil with a carrier. Apply to wrists.

Pleasing Bouquet: Create a citrus-floral scent by combining 8 drops of ylang-ylang with 8 drops of any two of the following: bergamot orange, geranium, grapefruit, lemon, marjoram, or vetiver oil.

Yearning Hearts: Create a wistful, romantic scent with 8 drops rose oil, 6 drops lime, and 6 drops vetiver oil plus a carrier. Apply to wrists and throat.

Dark Secrets: This one could be dangerous . . . combine 8 drops orange oil, 8 drops ylang-ylang, and 6 drops cedarwood or sandalwood with carrier oil. Apply to all pulse points.

Pure Romance: This scent carries a touch of the exotic: combine 8 drops jasmine, 6 drops clove oil, and 4 drops vanilla extract with your carrier. Place on wrists and throat.

DIY: Creating a Balanced Fragrance

You should blend scents as you would any perfume, incorporating top notes (the initial scent), middle notes (weightier than top notes), and base notes (the rich, lingering final scent). The correct blending ratio is 3:2:1, with base notes getting the fewest drops. Here are some examples of oils you can mix and match.

- Top notes: cinnamon, peppermint, lemon, or orange.
  - Middle notes: melissa, rosemary, lavender, nutmeg, or tea tree.
  - Base notes: clove, jasmine, ginger, and vanilla.

THE POTENT POWER OF AROMATHERAPY

The concept of inhaling aromatic natural oils goes back to ancient China, but the practice was not truly refined until the early 1900s. In 1937 French chemist René-Maurice Gattefossé came up with the name "aromatherapy."

Aromatherapy contends that inhaled scents can have an effect on the mental state and, in some cases, on the physical body itself. The physical process that activates our sense of smell is quite efficient: airborne molecules are drawn into the nose, where they strike olfactory neurons (nerve cells). Nerve impulses travel to a pair of olfactory bulbs connected to the limbic system, the seat of memory and emotion. In this way we quickly become aware of a scent, sometimes something so evocative that we are overcome by the memories. Smell is estimated to be 10,000 times more sensitive than the other senses, so it should not be surprising that it is capable of stimulating positive or negative emotional responses. In fact, scientists have linked smell to both memory and emotion.

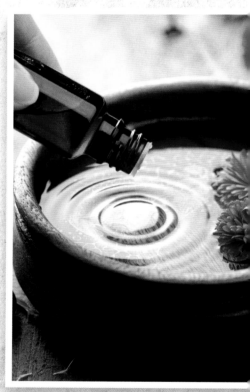

Essential oil for aromatherapy

A BRIEF HISTORY

The practice of inhaling aromatics to achieve spiritual connection occurred in many early civilizations, especially as part of religious rituals, but its roots as a mood enhancer probably began about 6,000 years ago in China. The Egyptians had a distillation process that separated the oils from plants such as clove, cedarwood, and cinnamon, which they then used for embalming. Hippocrates, the Greek "father of medicine," used herbal oils for healing purposes. After French chemist René-Maurice Gattefossé burned himself in a lab accident in 1910, he discovered the healing benefits of lavender oil and began exploring the healing potential of essential oils. When French surgeon Jean Valnet successfully used essential oils on wounded soldiers during World War I, he vindicated their medical benefits.

Today, aromatherapy is a large part of the wellness movement; it integrates nicely with bodywork therapy, such as massage and shiatsu, and has become part of the meditation process for many people. Some spas and resorts include aromatherapy sessions and teach aromatherapy classes.

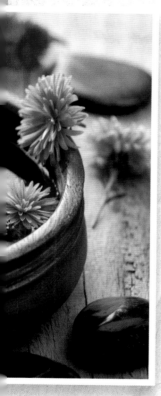

METHODS OF DELIVERY

Essential oils are traditionally accessed in a number of ways.

• Massage combines the hands-on benefits of bodywork with the therapeutic olfactory effects of the warm oils.

• Bathing with essential oils offers double benefits: the soothing effects of soaking in a warm tub, plus the healing, relaxing effects of the oils. Footbaths with essential oils are extremely restorative to tired, aching feet.

• Compresses allow essential oils to work on pain and stiffness. Simply apply 3 or 4 drops to a cold or hot compress and place it on the afflicted area.

• Steam inhalation requires filling a large bow with nearly boiling water, adding 3 or 4 drops of oil, and leaning over it with a towel draped over your head.

• The latest ultrasonic diffusers atomize the oils into the air without heat, helping to clear sinuses, coughs, or congestion.

FAMILIAL SCENTS

Familial scents aromatherapy incorporates a number of scent "families," which are based on aromas with similar attributes.

• Floral—rose, geranium, lavender, neroli, jasmine
• Woodsy—cedar, pine, sandalwood
• Earthy—vetiver, patchouli
• Citrus—orange, lemon, grapefruit, bergamot
• Herbaceous—rosemary, basil, clary sage
• Minty—peppermint, spearmint
• Camphorous—eucalyptus
• Spicy—cinnamon, clove, nutmeg
• Oriental—ginger

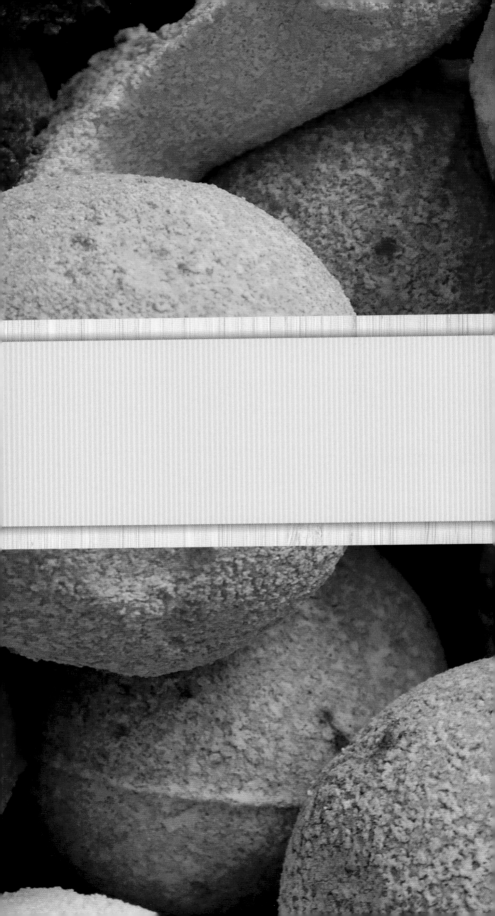

CHAPTER 5
NATURAL SPA TREATMENTS

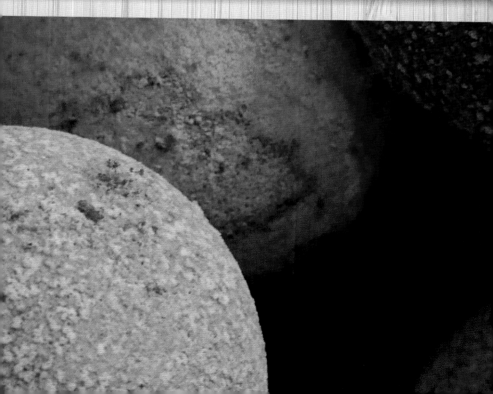

NATURAL SPA TREATMENTS

Spas have evolved from havens where the elite could go to rest and recuperate, to more health-oriented wellness centers that feature alternative options such as yoga. You can recapture the feeling of a spa at home not only by creating a serene space, but also by learning to make your own natural skin-, hair-, and nail-care products.

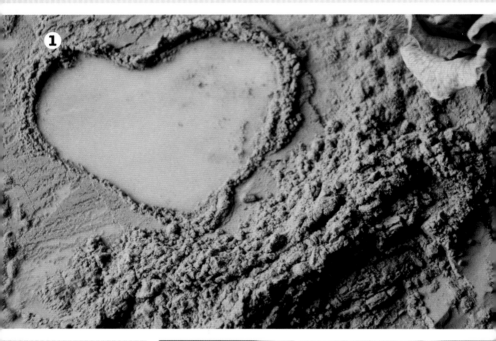

1 Healing
   minerals
2 Handmade soap
3 Kiwi mask
4 Salt crystals
5 Foot spa
6 Basic tool kit
   for making
   scrubs

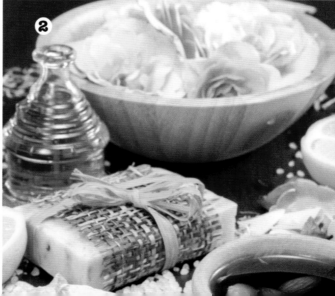

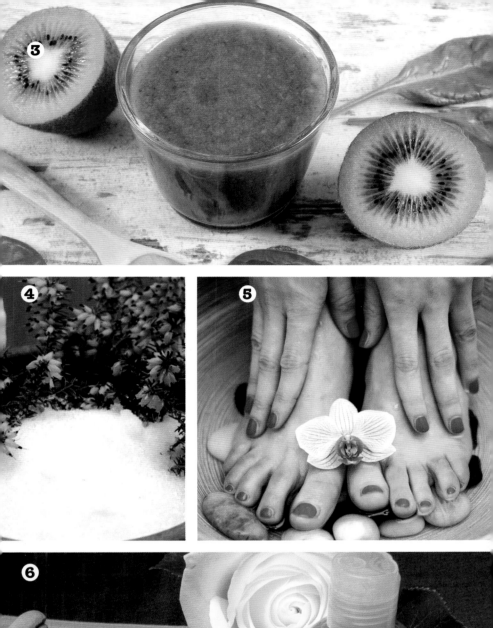

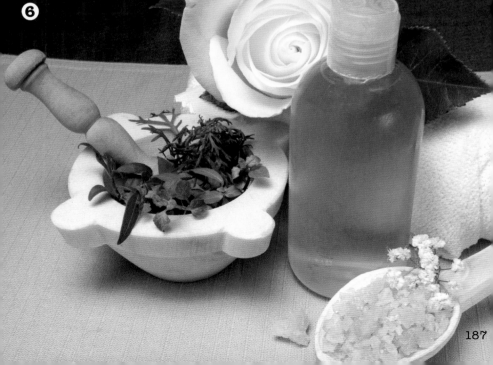

A HISTORY OF SPAS

Most women—and a surprising number of men—would agree that few things in life are as pleasurable as a restorative hour or two spent at a spa. But the concept of a spa has changed radically since the time of the great public baths of Greece and Rome.

It was the ancient cultures of the Mediterrean that popularized the concept of bathing for good health and mental uplift, creating elaborate bathhouses where politicians, citizens, and soldiers could get clean, have a massage, take steam, and gossip. The earliest true spas were created at locations with hot or cold springs, where people traveled to "take the waters," either by bathing in pools filled with mineral water to ease body aches or drinking the water as a tonic for the heart, lungs, gut, bowels, liver, reproductive organs, and kidneys. During the sixteenth century, the concept of bathing for improved health was revived in the English city of Bath, home to a famous hot spring and the remains of a Roman public bath. Around the same time a new location for drinking mineral water was created at a well in Yorkshire, a destination that became known as Harrogate.

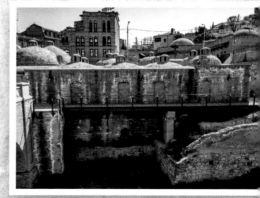

Sulfur baths in the ancient district of Tbilisi Abanotubani

Spas throughout Europe continued to cater to the wealthy and focus on the acts of bathing in and drinking the healing waters—although suitably ornate buildings were constructed to house these activities, and many amusing distractions such as gambling, horse races, and dances were offered. In the beginning of the twentieth century, strict diets and regimented exercise programs were added to the agenda at many spas. The emphasis shifted slightly from relaxing and taking the therapeutic waters to restoring the health—and waistlines—of overindulgent clients.

In America, the settlers learned the benefits of hot or mineral springs from Native Americans. The first commercial spa in the United States was at Saratoga Springs, New York, a city that hosted presidents, politicians, and the cream of society. Beauty or health spas became destinations for celebrities in the 1940s, when Hollywood stars and members of high society began flocking to these oases, where they could rest and refresh while enjoying first-class amenities and exploring many health treatments. These included mud baths, indoor and outdoor pools, steam rooms, saunas, several types of massage, electrolysis, juice or health bars, and weight rooms. Some celebrities visited spas to recuperate after plastic surgery; others rested up after detox programs. But most simply went to enjoy the feeling of being pampered in style while improving their health and their looks.

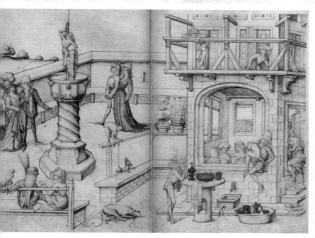

A bathhouse, c. 1475–1485

Today's modern spas are no longer based at mineral springs, but are more likely to be found in a mini-mall. They have, however, kept many of the principles of those early versions—treat patrons well and offer them a respite from the stresses of daily life. But they have also added more wellness treatments, though there are probably just as many beauty options. Modern menus may include manicures, pedicures, body waxing, bikini waxing, eyebrow waxing or stringing, massage, mud baths, whirlpools, seaweed wraps, facials, and weight-loss regimens. Some spas offer more new age choices, such as yoga, meditation, reflexology, acupuncture, hot stone massage, crystal therapy, and even sensory deprivation tanks, where you can float in meditative bliss for an hour or so.

Yet even at the most exclusive spas, many of the creams, lotions, and other skin-care treatments are commercial products that contain additives such as formaldehyde, coal tar, boric acid, phthalates, mercury, and sulfates, and preservatives such as parabens. You can replicate the spa experience right in your own home, but be sure to opt for nature-based treatments you prepare yourself from pantry items and essential oils.

HEALING WATERS:

Some historians believe the term "spa" comes from the Belgian town of Spa, which was lauded since Roman times for its healing mineral springs and at that time became known as Aquae Spadane. Others believe the name derives from the Latin phrase *salus per aquae*, or "health from water."

CREATE THE ULTIMATE HOME SPA

Imagine having a space in your home where you can kick back, relax, and let your skin-care products work their magic; where you can give yourself a manicure, a hot oil treatment, or an exfoliating foot massage—undisturbed.

To most people it's just the bathroom, but with the right touches, you can turn that cold, utilitarian space into a warm, soothing oasis, where you, your spouse, and even your kids will feel welcomed and pampered. All it takes is changing some paint colors and adding some decorating touches.

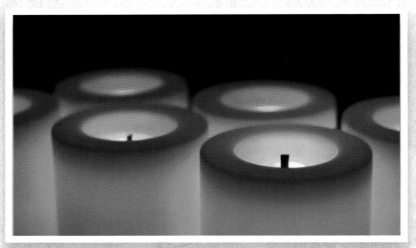

It is important to set the right mood

FIND THE RIGHT SHADE

Many older bathrooms have wall tiling that goes up to chair-rail height, leaving limited space for wall treatments. Plus, whatever color the tiling is, that's the color you're stuck with—we're not recommending a $10,000 bathroom renovation here. Fortunately, it's not hard to tone down your existing tile color. With yellow or peach tile, a pale bluish gray on the walls should work. Tone down green tiles with putty, oyster, or pale mushroom; tone down pinks with cool grays; and downplay brown tones with icy lavenders. If you have neutral beige, cream, or gray tiles, you can paint the walls any restful shade or indulge in designer wallpaper. To enhance your new walls, keep your task lighting over the sink and vanity mirror but provide softer lighting in the area of the bath or shower.

GATHER UP SUPPLIES

If space allows, add a wire or wooden standing rack to hold your bath and beauty supplies and folded towels. Otherwise hang up a roomy wall rack. You will need enough space to store all your toiletries and electronic grooming aids. Stock up on travel-sized bath and grooming products and consider purchasing stylish baskets or fabric bins to contain them all neatly.

ACCESSORIZE

Once you've prepared the room, it's time to add linens and some décor to personalize the space and augment the feeling of understated luxury. Don't forget to supply some music (safely away from water sources), flameless candles in different sizes, and a source of scent, such as an aromatherapy diffuser.

Shower curtain: This is the largest visual item in a bathroom; even when it's drawn closed, it makes a statement. A solid-colored curtain should not match your tile or walls, but be in the same family as one of them: for pale mint walls, use a medium teal curtain; for peach wall tiles, a terra cotta curtain. If you chosoe a print or pattern, make sure it is reflects your theme of inviting relaxation.

Worthy Towels: A spa is only as good as its towels, and your new space deserves 100 percent cotton. Purchase towel sets in shades that coordinate with your new color scheme. Add a few bath sheets to wrap yourself in Roman toga splendor. A plush or chenille bathroom rug is also a must. When drying your towels, omit the softening drier sheets—they affect absorbency.

Inflatable Neck Pillows: These are indispensable for those long soaks in scented bathwater.

Relaxing Artwork: Look for small, framed prints that reflect your idea of serenity or beauty. Black-and-white photographs can also be soothing, as can Chinese or Japanese brushwork or paintings.

Egg Timer: Warn the family that you are setting the timer for one hour, so you can achieve full relaxation. Soak in a tub scented with essential oils; give yourself a facial; pluck your eyebrows. Think mellow thoughts.

ASSESSING YOUR SKIN'S NEEDS

Once you have the right tools and ingredients, you can create your own nature-based creams, lotions, masks, toners, and scrubs—products that are custom made for your skin's specific requirements.

Before you begin preparing your own skin-care treatments, you need to determine what sort of skin you have. People generally have one of four types: dry, oily, combination, and normal. Excessively dry skin, also known as xerosis, can be sensitive, flaky, scaly, rough, red, itchy, sagging, or tired looking. Dry skin can be caused by cold weather, wind, central heating, overcleansing, aging, and disease. People deficient in essential nutrients such as beta-carotene, the B-complex vitamins, and vitamins C and E often suffer from dry skin.

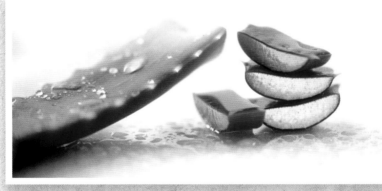

Sliced aloe vera

Oily skin is cause by excess sebum production; the complexion will be shiny and often experiences breakouts. Even people who think they have normal skin may have oily spots in the oil-gland-heavy T-zone, made up of the forehead, nose, and chin. This is combination skin and it may require two types of treatment.

THE pH FACTOR

Human skin has a light protective layer called the acid mantle. It is composed of sebum—free fatty acids—that mixes with lactic and amino acids from sweat to create a pH reading of about 5.5. This is the level that supports beneficial facial flora. (On the pH scale, 1 is the most acidic, 14 is the most alkaline.) If the skin's pH is not in balance due

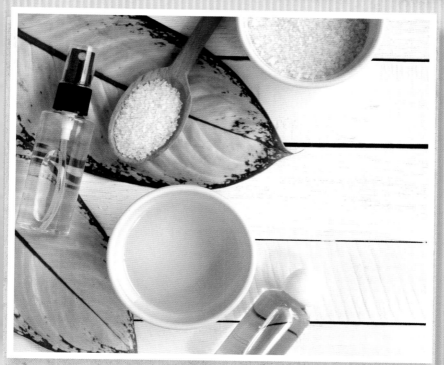

Natural skincare products, aromatherapy oil, and salt

to diet, skin products, smoking, air or water pollution, or too much sun, the result can be acne breakouts, infections, and even wrinkles. Most commercial soaps and cleansers are too alkaline, stripping away natural oils. Some ingredients, such as alpha hydroxy acids and retinoic acids, can be too acidic, weakening the skin's defenses against bacteria. You can apply topical antioxidants such as vitamins A, C, and E and green tea that help maintain the acid mantle, just don't use vitamin C with other acidic products. Aging skin also experiences a decrease in oil production. This can be rectified by masks based on olive, jojoba, argan, or coconut oils.

By creating skin-care products at home, you can be assured that your skin will be getting the appropriate cleansers, toners, and lotions for your precise complexion needs.

TOOL KIT SUGGESTIONS:

For preparing your own beauty products, you will need the items listed below. Keep all the smaller items together in a basket or bin.

• A number of small lidded glass jars (baby food jars are ideal)
• 3 or 4 lidded mason jars
• A plastic medicine dropper
• Measuring cups and measuring spoons
• Mixing bowls in several sizes
• Carrier oils such as olive, almond, and coconut
• A double boiler or two pots that create the same effect
• A supply of your favorite essential oils as well as some medicinal standbys, such as lavender, lemon balm, rosemary, and tea tree oil

FACIAL CLEANSERS

Whether you need a basic facial cleansing lotion or something more specific—for relieving acne, say, or deep cleaning grimy hands—creating custom cleansers should be well within your scope.

Our skin is exposed to so many pollutants in the course of each day, yet many of us omit a nightly cleaning ritual and then wonder why our skin looks patchy, lifeless, irritated, greasy, or red the next morning, or has begun breaking out. Plus too many commercial cleansing products, with all their chemical additives, may actually make matters worse. But with handmade cleansers you have the advantage of knowing exactly what went into them—only safe, natural ingredients.

ALL-PURPOSE CLEANSERS

These will be your everyday facial washes: easy to prepare, easy to apply, and mild but effective.

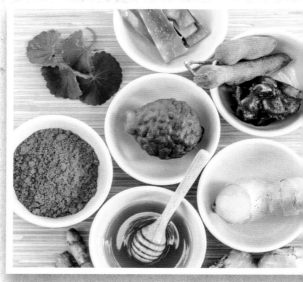

Homemade natural facial toner

Kitchen Choices:

To keep things really simple, there are pantry or refrigerator items you can use alone to clean your face, including honey, yogurt, olive oil, avocado, or pureed macadamia nuts. That latter two are rich in fatty acids and polyphenols that nourish the skin and combat signs of aging. Massage a light layer of the substance into your skin with a circular motion, then place a warm washcloth over your face to open the pores. Rinse with warm water.

Basic Skin Cleanser:

This standard recipe can be modified by changing up the essential oils. Begin with ¼ cup liquid castile soap combined with ¼ cup chamomile tea, and ¾ cup almond or olive oil, and add 8 drops of essential oil, your choice.

SPECIFIC REMEDIES:

You can also prepare cleansers to treat skin diseases or chronic conditions, reduce the signs of aging, remove grime, and slough off dead skin.

Skin Therapy: A soothing tisane made from fresh or dried chamomile steeped in hot water is ideal for bathing skin irritations, rashes, chicken pox, eczema, psoriasis, or sunburn. Dip a small cloth compress into comfortably hot tea and press against the affected area until the cloth cools. Repeat every four hours.

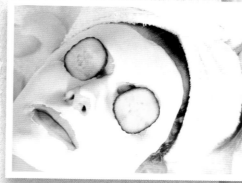

Face mask

Antiaging Cleanser: To prepare an effective antiaging facial cleanser, combine a tablespoon of aloe gel with a teaspoon of coconut oil, massage the mixture in your palms until it's warm, then use it to wash your face. Rinse and pat dry.

Handy Scrub: To fully clean greasy, grimy, or garden-soiled hands—or to exfoliate hands and feet while you're in the bath—combine a few drops of eucalyptus oil with Epsom salts and sea salt and use as a scrub.

ACNE TREATMENTS

Acne is generally caused by hormonal changes or fluctuations, but there are still steps you can take to prevent breakouts or heal them quickly.

Vanilla Acne Cure: Vanilla's antibacterial properties and healing B vitamins are able to combat flare-ups of acne and even reduce scarring from earlier outbreaks. Combine 5 drops of vanilla extract with 1 teaspoon honey and 1 teaspoon yogurt in a small bowl. Massage onto the face and leave on for 15 minutes before rinsing.

Acne Control: To prepare a gentle acne control that can also be used to remove makeup, mix ¼ cup canola oil with 10 drops tea tree oil in a small, lidded glass jar and shake well. Apply to outbreaks with a cotton ball or swab, rinse with warm water, and end with a mild toner.

Face sponges

MAKE YOUR OWN SOAPS

Imagine your spa space decorated with beneficial herbal soaps in a variety of shapes, colors, and scents that you created yourself. They also make wonderful hostess gifts or additions to gift baskets.

Soap making goes back at least to 2800 BC, to ancient Babylon, where inscriptions were found on a soap container that advised boiling fats with ashes, similar to the methods used today. Wood ashes contain lye, a highly caustic substance that converts fats or oils into cleansing agents during a chemical reaction called saponification.

THE MELT-AND-MOLD METHOD

Although it is almost impossible to make soap from scratch without using lye, the recipes presented here use premade bar soaps that already contain lye, so you don't have to measure it out or handle it at all. These recipes employ the melt-and-mold method, not the complex hot-process method. You will naturally want to add essential oils, but also consider including food coloring, and ground oatmeal or dried herbs and flowers for texture. You can order different styles of silicon soap molds online, or simply use a muffin tin or mini bundt pan.

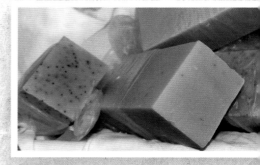

Basic Recipe: Grate 8 ounces of glycerin, castile, goat's milk, or any other natural soap and melt it in the top of a double boiler, stirring slowly. Add ingredients such as food

Handmade soap

coloring, herbs, flowers, or exfoliants such as oatmeal, ground walnuts, or almonds. You can also add an ounce or two of green tea, brewed coffee, coconut milk, or floral hydrosol. Take the mixture off the heat and add 5 to 10 drops of essential oils. When the mixture is blended, pour into soap molds or muffin tins. Wait 30 minutes for the surface to harden, then place containers in the freezer for 20 minutes, until soap is firm and cool. Unmold soaps onto a dish towel and allow them to dry an additional two days.

To Add Herbs or Flowers: Boil ¼ cup water, add 2 to 4 teaspoons of ground, dried botanicals, and let them steep for 15 minutes.

Holiday Bounty: This seasonally scented soap makes a great stocking stuffer. Arrange a mixture of dried hibiscus, juniper berries, lemon peel, rose petals, and eucalyptus in the molds. Then combine clear glycerin soap with essential oils such as eucalyptus, lemon, orange, and rosemary and pour into the molds. When dry, store soaps in airtight containers.

Healing Charcoal Soap: Activated charcoal is a detoxifying exfoliant, so this blend works well on acne-prone skin. Begin with ½ pound of cubed shea butter soap; once it has melted, take a small amount and stir in 5 capsules of activated charcoal or 1 teaspoon of powder before returning mixture to the pot. Remove from heat, add 10 or 15 drops of tea tree oil (peppermint works well, too), and stir.

Coffee-Cinnamon Scrub Soap: Coffee grounds provide the exfoliating factor here and cinnamon adds a spicy note. Use ½ pound of castile soap in your basic recipe and add 1 teaspoon of coffee grounds and 5 to 8 drops of cinnamon oil. You can even tint the soap with the addition of an ounce of brewed coffee.

Lavender & Honey Soap: Adorn this soap with a few sprigs of lavender tied on with a hemp cord and give as Easter or Mother's Day gifts. Start by melting 2 pounds of goat's milk soap (makes 6–8 bars), adding the zest of 1 lemon, 3 tablespoons of dried lavender buds, 15 drops lavender oil, 6 drops lemon oil, and 2 tablespoons honey.

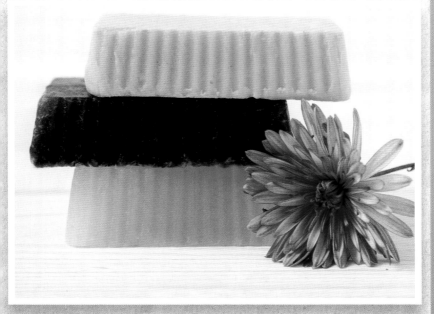

Natural handmade soap

TONERS AND ASTRINGENTS

Once your face has been thoroughly cleansed and before you apply a moisturizer, you will want to use a toner to lock in moisture and shrink the pores. Even dry skin can benefit from a gentle toner every few days.

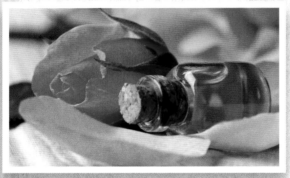

Rose water

TIGHTEN UP

Toners, also called astringents, can not only cleanse and reduce the size of pores, prevent breakouts, and regulate sebum production, they also balance the skin's pH and help it heal.

The easiest way to apply liquid toner is with a cotton ball or makeup square; that way it won't end up running down your forehead into your eyes. Or place the toner in a spray bottle and give your face a gentle spritz. Keep toners in the refrigerator for an extra-refreshing experience.

Top Tea Toner: This beneficial recipe offers antioxidant, astringent, antibacterial, and antiviral properties. Combine ¾ cup brewed green tea (made with 3 tea bags) and ¼ cup apple cider vinegar. Pour into a jar or bottle, add 5 drops tea tree essential oil (or any preferred oil), and shake well. This keeps for a week in the refrigerator. Avoid eyes when applying.

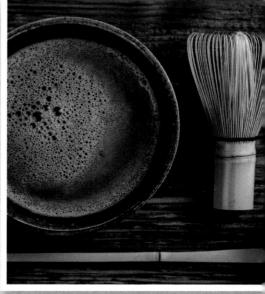

Green tea matcha

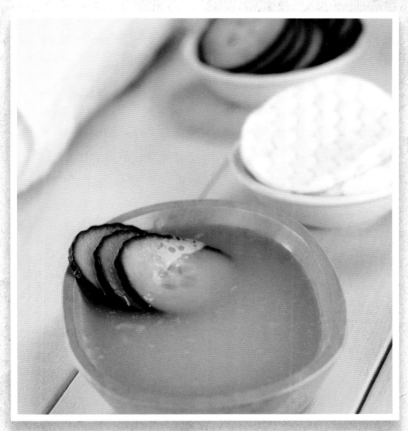

Homemade natural cucumber facial toner

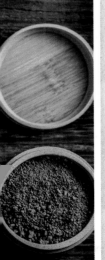

Hydrating Herbal Toner: Begin with 3 tablespoons rose water, 2 tablespoons witch hazel, 1 teaspoon apple cider vinegar, 8 drops rose hip oil, 4 drops tea tree oil, and 5 drops lavender or other herbal essential oil. Place the ingredients in a small bowl and whisk them together. Pour into a glass spray bottle. To use, close your eyes and spray your face, lightly massaging the toner into the skin. Follow with a moisturizer. It can also be used to refresh skin before bedtime.

Honey Pore Cleanser: Honey contains enzymes that are able to clarify the skin and clear the pores, leaving skin with a more even tone. Combine 2 tablespoons coconut oil with 1 tablespoon honey and apply the mixture to clean, dry skin (avoiding the eyes). Then rinse.

Vinegar Toner: Using vinegar to tighten pores supposedly goes back to Helen of Troy. Mix 1 tablespoon apple cider vinegar with 2 cups of cool water and use as an astringent finisher to clean and tighten your skin and restore your acid mantle.

GENTLE FACIAL MASKS

Many facial beauty products include aloe vera gel. To access the gel from a plant, simply break off a leaf, slice it down the center with a knife and harvest the beneficial gel with its antioxidant healing properties.

RESTORE YOUR COMPLEXION

Moisturizing masks that return hydration to facial skin and help reduce the look of wrinkles, sagging, and broken capillaries should become part of your weekly beauty regimen.

Aloe for Sensitive Skin: Aloe vera can be used as a non-greasy makeup remover, but with its antibacterial properties it also makes a superior face mask for those who have sensitive skin, acne, or rosacea. Mix a tablespoon of fresh aloe gel with a teaspoon of almond milk and a teaspoon of lemon juice. Pat onto your face, leave on for three minutes, then rinse.

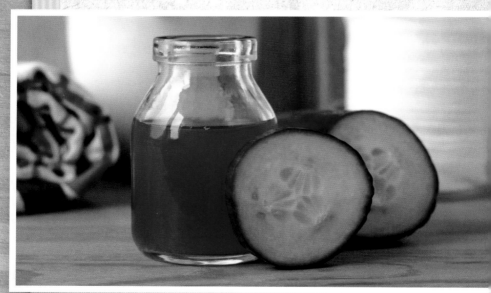

Cucumber juice in a small glass jar for preparing facial toner

Cumin Care: For exfoliated, radiant skin, create a mask made of one part turmeric to three parts cumin blended into honey or yogurt. Apply to the face and leave on until it dries.

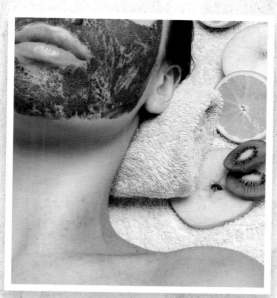

Natural homemade fruit facial masks

Vitality Masks: For a mask that will wake up your face, combine 1 teaspoon plain yogurt, the juice from an orange quarter along with some pulp, and 1 teaspoon aloe gel. Keep the mixture on for 5 minutes before rinsing. Or try a revitalizing mask of mild yellow mustard left on for a minute or two. Test a small skin patch for irritation first. Or mix the juice from one lemon with ¼ cup olive or almond oil.

Oatmeal Complexion Calmer: Combine ½ cup of hot water with ⅓ cup of oatmeal and let it steep for a few minutes. Then mix in 2 tablespoons plain yogurt, 2 tablespoons honey, and one egg white. Apply thinly to the face and wait 10 minutes. Rinse with warm water.

Puffy Eye Rx: A quick fix for inflamed, dry, or irritated eyes is soaking two tea bags in warm water for 10 minutes, squeezing out excess moisture, and pressing them over your eyes. Or place a cucumber slice under each eye to hydrate the delicate tissues.

More Solutions: There are many items right in your home that can make effective masks, including mayonnaise, coconut oil, olive oil, witch hazel, cucumber juice, green tea, and wheat germ oil. An easy mayo mask involves applying it straight to the face, leaving it on for 20 minutes. After a thorough rinsing, your skin will feel baby soft.

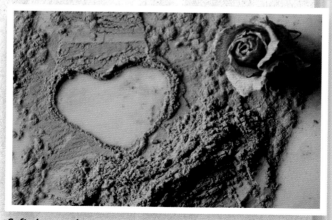

Soft clay powder

EXFOLIANTS AND SCRUBS

Combining a carrier oil with a mild abrasive to remove dead skin cells not only leaves your complexion polished and glowing, it can reduce acne breakouts. For best results, use carriers such as olive, almond, argan, or coconut oil.

SIMPLE AND SWEET

Sugar is a pantry staple that makes an excellent facial abrasive. Overuse of facial scrubs, however, can be hard on delicate tissues, so unless your skin gets a build up of dead cells, restrict exfoliating sessions to once a week. Be careful to avoid the eyes and the sensitive skin below them when applying any type of abrasive. You should also moisturize soon after removing the scrub.

Basic Sugar Scrub: Combine 1 teaspoon granulated sugar, 2 drops of water, and a few drops of orange, lemon, or lavender essential oil. Gently massage into face, being careful to avoid the eyes. Rinse with cool water and pat dry.

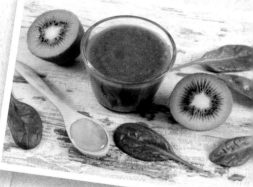

Quick Sugar Scrub:
Combine ¼ cup of coconut oil and 1

Kiwi and honey

tablespoon of granulated sugar in a small bowl, and stir well. With gentle, circular motions, massage the scrub into clean facial and neck skin for 60 seconds. Rinse with warm water. This scrub also makes an effective exfoliant to use before shaving if you want smooth, silky legs when summer weather approaches.

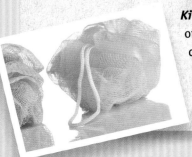

Kiwi Honey Scrub: Combine ¼ cup of kiwi (or other soft fruit), 2 teaspoons honey, and 1 or 2 tablespoons sugar. Mix in blender until smooth, then place a thin layer on your face, and leave on for 15 minutes. Rinse with warm water.

Cinnamon Scrub: When used as a scrub, this spice produces a clear, radiant complexion. Combine ½ cup almond oil with 1 teaspoon cinnamon, and massage into face and neck. Rinse and pat dry.

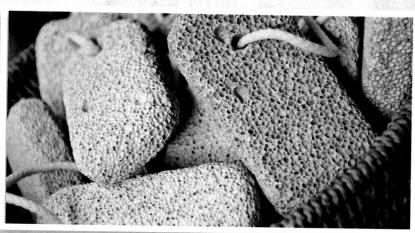

Colorful pumices in a basket

Walnut Scrub: Most coarse-ground nuts make effective exfoliants. Combine a teaspoon of ground walnuts to ½ cup yogurt and 1 teaspoon honey and massage gently into the face. Rinse with warm water. It also works as a body scrub in the shower. Other variations include adding the walnuts to ⅛ cup of olive or coconut oil, or combining them with half a pureed avocado.

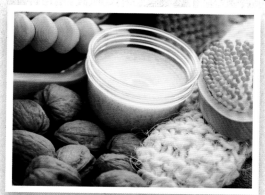

Walnut scrub

Parsley-Walnut Scrub: Start with a bunch of parsley, chop it fine, and steep it in a bowl of boiling water for 10 or 15 minutes. Strain the cooled parsley and muddle it into 1 teaspoon ground walnut and one teaspoon fuller's earth. Massage the mask gently onto your face and leave it on until it dries. Splash you face with warm water and massage skin again. Rinse off with warm water. Moisturize immediately.

DIY: The Salt Method

Sea salt can also be used as an exfoliant, although the particles tend to be larger than sugar grains, therefore more abrasive. You may want to reserve salt scrubs for use on the body. A basic formula for creating a salt scrub is 1 cup fine ground sea salt, ¼ cup carrier oil, and 10 drops of your favorite aromatic or healing essential oil. Consider sandalwood, patchouli, or rosemary oils, or a citrus blend.

FACIAL MOISTURIZERS

Our facial skin puts up with a lot of stressors—makeup; loss of sleep; alcohol; the heat from hair dryers; cold, windy winters; dry central heating; and pollution. So give your face a replenishing treat at least once a day.

FACE FORWARD:

The point of moisturizing is not just to relieve dry skin. Hydrating the skin properly with natural ingredients also provides key nutrients to enhance the skin and leave it more elastic and resilient. Many of the ingredients in the moisturizers below are items you already have in your refrigerator or pantry.

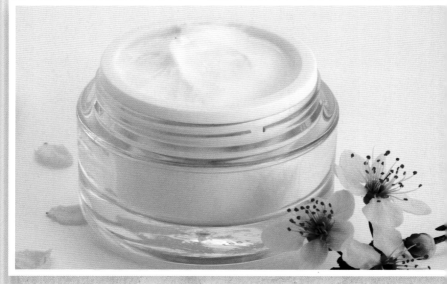

Facial moisturizer

Vitamin C Brightener: This treatment provides a fresh glow to tired-looking skin. Start with 1 teaspoon vitamin C powder, 1 teaspoon spring water, 1½ tablespoons aloe vera gel, 1 teaspoon vitamin E oil, and 5 drops frankincense essential oil. Briskly blend vitamin C powder with water, then add aloe and blend again. Then mix in all other ingredients. Place liquid in a small, colored bottle to reduce light deterioration. Massage onto your face every other night, but be sure to remove it in the morning—vitamin C can cause sensitivity to sunlight.

Therapeutic Lip Balm: To make a healing balm for chapped skin or lips, combine 5 tablespoons Saint-John's-wort oil with 2 teaspoons beeswax in the top of a double boiler. Add 3 drops vitamin E oil and 5 drops of an essential oil. Melt over heat, then quickly transfer the mixture to a covered tin or container before it thickens.

Egg Facial: To alleviate dry skin, beat an egg yolk lightly and apply it to the face. Wait 30 minutes before rinsing. Your skin will be fresh and supple. For oily skin, use only the egg white; use the entire egg on normal skin.

Banana Mash: For a rejuvenating treatment, mash up a small banana and blend it with ¼ cup plain yogurt and 2 tablespoons honey. Apply the mixture to your face and neckline and wait 20 minutes before rinsing with cold water.

The Lush Touch: This recipe does require several essential oils, but it may be the ultimate face softener. You will need 3 ounces argan oil, 1 ounce shea butter, 1 ounce carrot seed oil, 5 drops lemongrass oil, 10 drops lavender oil, and 6 drops chamomile oil. Place the argan and shea oil in a glass or aluminum bowl and place the bowl in a pan of warm water. Once the shea butter has melted, blend the two oils. Add the carrot oil and blend, then add the remaining oils and blend again. Store in a glass jar in a cool dark place.

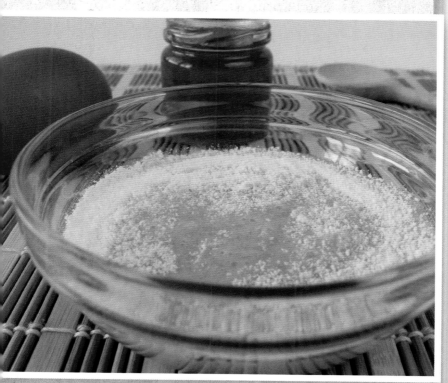

Face mask with honey, egg yolk, and powdered milk

HEALING HONEY TREATMENTS

Honey is one of those miracle foods—used as a sweetener for eons, it doesn't go bad, and its antioxidant and antiseptic properties provide impressive health benefits. Plus, it's just so natural—made by honeybees from plant nectar.

YOUR SKIN'S BEST FRIEND
Because honey has a virtually limitless shelf life, it's something many of us keep around the house, sometimes for years. So take that old jar of honey from the pantry and repurpose it as your skin's new best friend. It soothes, smoothes, diminishes scars, and even reduces signs of aging.

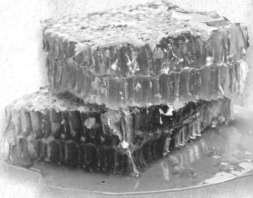

Honeycomb

Honey-Oatmeal Acne Scrub: This simple exfoliating face scrub can moisturize, even out skin tone, and may help to reduce breakouts. Combine ½ cup uncooked oats, 2 tablespoons honey, 1 teaspoon nutmeg, 10 drops lavender essential oil, 10 drops tea tree essential oil, and 1 teaspoon dried lavender. Massage into face for several minutes and then rinse with cool water.

Honey-Milk Moisture Mask: Honey is both emollient and hydrating, even when used on its own as a mask. For a more penetrating treatment, mix together 1 tablespoon buttermilk, 1 teaspoon honey, and 1 egg yolk, then apply to the face (avoiding the eyes) and leave on for 15 minutes.

Honey Citrus Mask: This preparation combines the antioxidant and antibacterial power of honey with the exfoliating and acne-fighting properties of the citric acid found in lemons. Combine 2 teaspoons honey with 1 teaspoon fresh lemon juice. Massage the mixture between your fingers until it warms up, then apply a thin layer to your face and neck. Let the mask dry and then rinse with warm water.

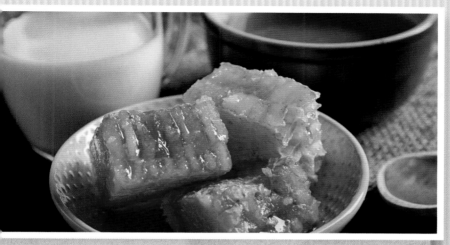

Milk and honey

Sweet Soak: Cleopatra's favorite beauty secret will leave your body baby soft. Combine ¼ cup honey with 2 cups milk and add a few drops of essential oil. Stir and add to your bath water. A little baking soda will also help soften skin.

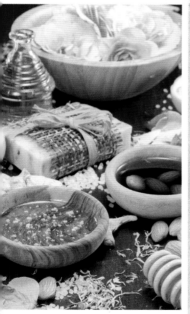

Honey, citrus fruit, and almonds

Moisturizing Body Mask: Combine 1 tablespoon of honey with 1 tablespoon of olive oil and a dash of lemon juice and apply to elbows, knees, heels, and any other dry, flaky body parts. Leave on for 20 minutes; rinse well afterward.

Honey-Almond Scrub: This is a great body scrub for any time of year. Add 3 tablespoons ground almonds to 2 tablespoons of honey and use the paste to exfoliate your skin in the shower.

Scar Treatment: Honey can lighten skin and help regenerate the tissue on scars. Mix 1 teaspoon raw honey with 1 teaspoon coconut oil, apply it to scar and then cover with a hot wash cloth. Remove when cool. This can be repeated daily.

Sun Saver: Combine 1 part honey with 2 parts aloe vera gel for a healing, hydrating treatment for sunburned skin.

SHAMPOO ENHANCER:
You can add honey to your shampoo to strengthen hair and help it retain moisture. Squeeze some shampoo into a small bowl and add 1 teaspoon of honey. Blend the two liquids slowly until the thicker honey "melts" into the shampoo, then use on your hair as you normally would.

CALMING OATMEAL CURES

Oatmeal is so naturally soothing to the skin that it is often added to anti-itch lotions, cleansers, and shampoos. When coarsely ground, it also acts as an exfoliant. Use only whole raw oats, not instant oatmeal, in skin-care recipes.

REDUCE INFLAMMATION

Oatmeal contains natural emollients, which is why it should be your first choice when it comes to easing skin irritation. It not only cleanses and moisturizes, it also combats dryness by creating a protective layer that augments the skin's normal barrier function. So the next time your skin feels tight, swollen, or scratchy, let the calming effects of oatmeal remove puffiness and inflammation from your face and body.

Oatmeal Beauty Mask: This rich formula will give you flawless skin. In a dish, combine ¼ cup warm spring water with 1 teaspoon coconut oil, then gradually stir in 3 tablespoons raw oats. Mix into a paste, apply to face and neck, and leave on for 10 minutes. Rinse with warm water.

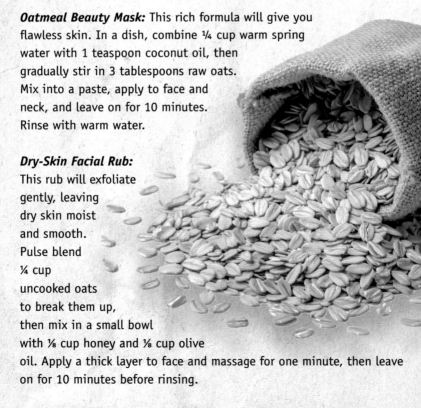

Dry-Skin Facial Rub: This rub will exfoliate gently, leaving dry skin moist and smooth. Pulse blend ¼ cup uncooked oats to break them up, then mix in a small bowl with ⅛ cup honey and ⅛ cup olive oil. Apply a thick layer to face and massage for one minute, then leave on for 10 minutes before rinsing.

Oatmeal Soak: This bath treatment can ease the itching of dry skin, dermatitis, eczema, sunburn, insect bites, hives, and poison ivy. Finely

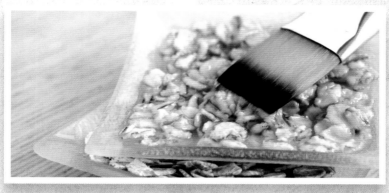

Homemade oatmeal mask

grind a cup of raw oats in a blender and pour it into the tub as you run a warm bath. Blend well before entering the tub, then lie back and relax for 15 to 30 minutes. This bath recipe can also be safely used on dogs suffering from flea bites, hot spots, or seasonal itching. For an additional soothing scent, add 10 drops of chamomile and lavender oil. Whole oats can be placed in the toe of a knee-high stocking; knot it, and swirl it in the tub.

Soothing Eczema Soak: This bath additive is intended to relieve the relentless itching of eczema. Combine 3 tablespoons extra-virgin olive oil with ¼ cup baking soda and ½ cup finely ground oats. Mix the ingredients with your bathwater and soak for at least 20 minutes.

During colder weather when eczema flares up, this routine should probably be repeated once a week.

Junior Version: Create a safe treatment for infants or toddlers who suffer from eczema by mixing 3 teaspoons olive oil, 1 tablespoon baking soda, and 2 tablespoons oats in a baby-sized tub of warm water. Let baby soak until the water cools.

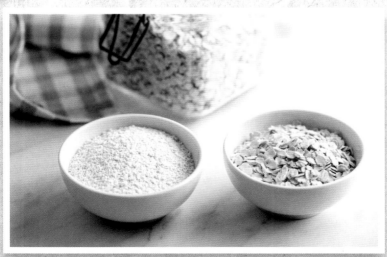

Dry rolled and ground oatmeal in bowls

MAKE YOUR OWN BATH OILS

There are few things as indulgent as taking a long, soaking bath. And when you add essential oils, with their relaxing scents and medicinal benefits, your bath becomes a therapeutic experience as well.

By using essential oils and other botanicals in your bath, you can transform a humdrum soak into a truly relaxing respite from stress, aggravation, and your daily worries. As heated water carries the calming or reviving scents through the air, you will feel the outer world recede, allowing you to focus on you.

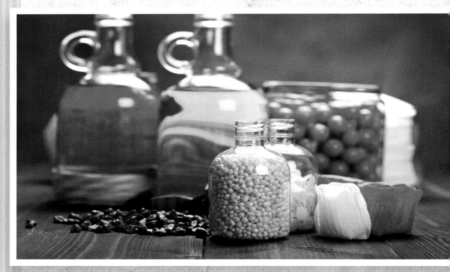

Bath salt and oils

CUSTOM SCENTS

By carefully choosing which essential oil or oils you add to your bath, you can alter the end result. You may need to ease tension one day, be energized the next. Experiment not only with mixing the oils, but with determining how many drops you need to add to achieve the perfect ambiance.

Calming Oils: Tone things down with bee balm, lavender, vanilla, ginger, and nutmeg.

Healthiest Oils: For a straight-up therapeutic bath, try any of the following oils: clove, eucalyptus, frankincense, lavender, chamomile, lemon, oregano, peppermint, rosemary, and sage.

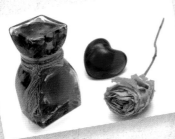

Child-safe Bath Additives: Because young children often get bathwater in their mouths, it's best not to use essential oils in their bath. Opt instead for zesty lemon juice, soothing baking soda, or pH-restoring apple cider vinegar.

Refreshing and Uplifting Oils: Regain energy and renew insight with eucalyptus, peppermint, rosemary, fennel, bergamot orange, lemon balm, clary sage, and juniper.

Herbal Notes: For a truly earthy, herbal scent that's made for outdoorsy types, try mixing 10 drops of lavender essential oil, 5 drops of frankincense oil, and 3 drops of cedarwood oil with ½ cup of carrier oil.

Citrus Soak: Perk up your skin and your senses by combining the scents of several oils in the citrus family: grapefruit, orange, mandarin, lemon, and bergamot orange.

Sensual Scents: Prepare for a romantic night on the town—or an evening in—with the oils of coriander, patchouli, vanilla, or aniseed.

Luxurious Moments: Pretend you are an Arabian Nights princess or a film noir femme fatale as you surround yourself with the rich scents of jasmine, tuberose, ylang-ylang, neroli, or clary sage oil.

Masculine Essence: There's no reason women should get all the benefits from moisturizing bath oils. After all, men are more often asked to perform outdoor work that exposes their skin to the elements in all four seasons. For a manly yet restorative soak, try sandalwood, eucalyptus, bay, cypress, patchouli, ginger, black pepper, vanilla, vetiver, and any of the citrus oils. Or mix up a custom blend to your own taste.

REFRESHING DRINKS:
While you are relaxing in a warm tub, it makes a nice contrast to hydrate your insides by sipping a cool drink. Try adding sliced cucumbers or a few lemon or lime wedges and ice to spring water. Or turn a strong cup of brewed herbal tea into iced tea before you prepare the bath. Serve drinks in an insulated cup to keep them chilled.

BATH BOMBS AND FIZZIES

Who doesn't love a big, colorful, scented bath ball that fizzes wildly when you drop it into the tub? Bath bombs and fizzies have become the bath-time rage with both kids and adults, and they are incredibly easy to make.

These popular bath bombs can be costly in specialty bed-and-bath stores but they are relatively inexpensive to make. Most of the ingredients are found around the house, and the only real costs are a few essential oils and a dozen or so silicone molds, which are available on the internet. The bombs average out to about $2 apiece, less if you plan on making them in quantity. These fizzies are not only fun to use at home, they make terrific gifts—and can even be color or scent themed for different holidays.

BOMBS AWAY!
The following basic recipe makes 12 bombs, so be sure you've purchased enough molds to accommodate them. The batter hardens quickly, so you can't mold the bombs in smaller batches.

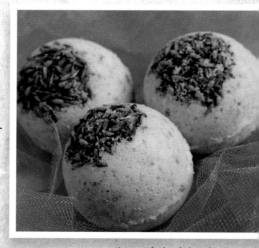
Aromatic bath bombs

Ingredients:

- 4 ounces Epsom salts
- 8 ounces baking soda
- 4 ounces cornstarch
- 4 ounces citric acid
- 2½ tablespoons coconut or olive oil
- 1 tablespoon water
- 2 teaspoons essential oil, your choice
- 4 to 6 drops of food coloring
- 12 to 18 silicone molds

In a large bowl mix the dry ingredients together so there are no clumps. Place the wet ingredients in a jar and shake them up. Add the liquid to the dry ingredients in slow, tiny increments. This is really critical—you don't want the mixture to start fizzing prematurely if the baking soda starts reacting to the citric acid. Stop blending and wait if fizzing begins. The finished mixture should just barely clump together. Now quickly press the mixture into the molds, because it will start to harden almost immediately. The bombs should take approximately one day to dry, a bit longer if your molds have intricate details. Test one bomb in the tub and watch it explode into colorful bubbles. Wrap each bomb in cellophane and prepare to hand them out, perhaps with a small tag describing their scent.

CUSTOMIZED SCENTS

You can add or mix essential oils so that the bombs give off different scents to match your tastes or to capture the essence of a time of year. Each batch should need about 2 teaspoons of essential oil, less if you choose to combine scents.

Holiday Scents: To capture the spirit of Thanksgiving or the winter holidays, try combining cinnamon oil with clove, cocoa with peppermint, coffee or nutmeg with vanilla, or cedar with any berry oil.

Summery Scents: Any lighter, "green" oils would work here, but especially lemon balm, lemon verbena, bergamot orange, bee balm, lavender, sage, or fennel in a blue-green bomb.

Autumn Scents: Capture the season of bonfires and spooky nights with licorice, sandalwood, cedar, cocoa, or juniper in an orange bomb.

Exotic Scents: Create a sense of allure with the oils of jasmine, vanilla, ylang-ylang, neroli, frankincense, myrrh, or patchouli, perhaps in medium purple or amber.

Spa Scent: Try combining the classic therapeutic scents of eucalyptus and lavender in a pastel-colored bath bomb.

Kid's Favorites: Since very little essential oil goes into the bathwater, these fizzies should be safe for children old enough not to get water in their mouths. Try blending essential oils to make "Creamsicle bombs" (vanilla and orange), "Fudgsicle bombs" (cocoa and vanilla), "lemon fizzes" (lemon oil and lavender), or "cinna-bombs" (using cinnamon, nutmeg, and vanilla oils). Kids also enjoy the addition of biodegradable glitter and dried flower petals. Don't forget to make some zany color combos, too.

EPSOM SALTS AND BATH SOAKS

Bath oils may moisturize the skin, but bath salts go deeper, removing damaging toxins from the body, as well as loosening stiff, aching joints. They are simple to prepare and can be scented to suit your mood.

The medicinal use of salt baths goes back at least to biblical times, probably well before that. In theory, Epsom salts break down in water to produce magnesium, a muscle relaxant, and sulfate, which clears toxins, and each enters the body through the skin. Toxins are poisonous or harmful substances—such as pollution, the chemicals in processed foods, and pesticides—that we come into contact with each day and that negatively affect us. So it makes sense that when you shed those toxins, your health will reflect the positive changes. Bath salts can also lower stress; soften skin; treat a tight, congested chest; and boost energy levels.

SOAK IMPURITIES AWAY
The following detoxifying bath recipes will give you a high-end spa experience for almost no cost.

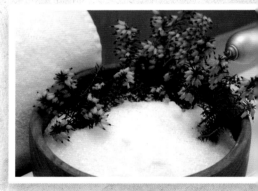

Bowl filled with Epsom salts

Basic Detox Salt Soak:
Combine ¼ cup sea salt or Himalayan salt, ¼ cup Epsom salt (to relieve tired muscles and reduce inflammation), ¼ cup baking soda (to soften skin and ease skin irritation), and add to your bathwater. You might also include ⅓ cup apple cider vinegar for its astringent and pH-balancing properties. You can increase the ingredients proportionally by 3 or 4 times so you will have premixed salts on hand for a week or two.

SCENT OPTIONS
To the basic recipe, you can add 8 to 10 drops of a favorite essential oil, or blend several to create a personalized scent. The inclusion of these oils provides anti-inflammatory, antimicrobial, and antioxidant benefits.

And don't forget to add appropriate food coloring to your salts, especially if you display them in clear glass or plastic containers— simply place the salts in a plastic bag with a few drops of coloring and shake vigorously to disperse the color.

Relaxation: For a soothing tension buster, try 4 drops each lavender and cedarwood or 4 drops each lavender and bergamot orange. Color the blend purple or orange or mix the two.

Wake-up Call: For a refreshing morning bath, try 3 drops of peppermint oil and 4 drops of ylang-ylang. Color the salts pink or peach.

Citrus Soaker: To the basic recipe, add 6 drops of grapefruit oil and 3 drops of lemon to amp up your levels of energy and happiness. Color the salts pink and yellow.

Sweet & Spicy: Mix eucalyptus oil with vanilla oil and add to the basic recipe for an unusual earthy combo that will act as a natural deodorant and soften skin. Color the salts greenish yellow.

Blemish Buster: Lemon oil is known to promote clean, clear skin; combine 4 drops lemon oil with 4 drops rosemary or eucalyptus oil and add to the salts recipe.

Back Bracer: After a strenuous workout at the gym or a taxing yoga session, give your back muscles some hydrotherapy—add 3 drops of peppermint oil and 4 of cinnamon oil to the salts recipe for quick relief.

Congestion Relief: There is nothing quite like breathing in eucalyptus vapors to ease the congestion of colds and flu. Add 5 drops eucalyptus oil and 4 drops clove, tea tree, or thyme oil to a comfortably hot bath.

Milk Bath: Combine ½ cup of Epsom salts with ½ cup of powdered milk, which will help slough off dead skin.

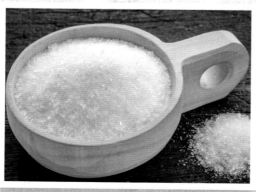

Honey-Almond Salts: Create this skin softener by combining ½ cup Epsom salts with 2 tablespoons of honey and 6 drops of almond essential oil. Color salts a deep amber.

Magnesium sulfate (Epsom salts)

HAND AND NAIL TREATMENTS

In most job situations, from the fast-food weekend gig to the executive suite, women and men need to have well-groomed hands. This level of care is not hard to attain, though, even without a visit to the local manicure parlor.

Our hands say a lot about us. Work-roughened hands, dirty or unkempt fingernails, or torn cuticles are not appealing. Wearing rings and bracelets also calls attention to hands and nails, so make sure yours are always presentable, even if it simply means moisturizing, filing, and the application of clear polish. Your feet, too, should never be so rough and callous, or have toenails so long and ragged.

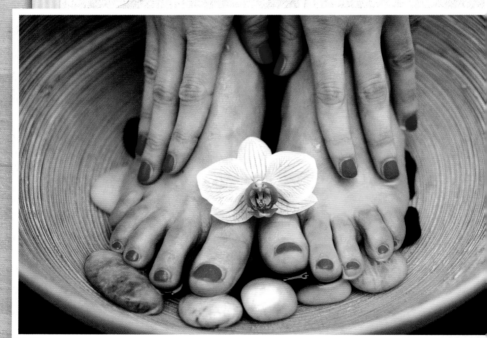

Female feet in spa bowl with sea salt

TRICKS AND TIPS

Below are some easy-to-follow treatments that will make sure you always leave the house with neat, attractive nails.

Hot Oil Hand Treatment: This simple trick will soften your hands and benefit your nails as well. Microwave ⅓ cup of extra-virgin olive oil for

20 seconds. Massage the oil into your hands and cuticles. Cover each hand in plastic wrap. Soak your hands in warm water for 5 minutes to help the oil absorb better.

Cuticle Creams: Healthy nails begin with smooth, healthy cuticles. Mix 1 or 2 ounces of beeswax pellets (available online), 3 ounces apricot kernel oil, and 1 tablespoon honey in a paper bowl. Heat for 15-second increments in a microwave until melted. Blend and place in a small lozenge tin. Or whip together 1 drop of your favorite essential oil with 2 tablespoons coconut oil, or an equal amount aloe vera gel and coconut oil, and store the cream in a small glass jar.

The Perfect Manicure: With practice you can handle nails like a pro. Soak fingertips in warm sudsy water, then dry. Gently push cuticles back with the flat end of an orange stick. Trim nails straight across then round the sides in a curve. File them smooth with a 4-way emery stick—use rough grade, fine grade, then buff. Apply base coat, moisturize your hands, add two light coats of polish, then finish with the top coat.

The Manly Manicure: Men who want well-groomed hands and nails should invest in a good nail clipper and several 4-way emery boards. Trim and even out the top edge of the nails, then apply a clear matte polish or simply polish the surface with the buffing side of the 4-way emery board. Apply olive oil or cuticle oil to fingertips at least twice a week.

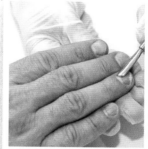

Male manicure

The Manly Pedicure: Far too many men feel free to wear sandals without really taking a good look at their rough toenails. If you have overgrown or ragged nails, it is the work of five minutes to correct them. First, clean your nails with a toothbrush. Then use the flat end of an orange stick to gently ease cuticles back. Use a large nail clipper to trim off excess nail—cut straight across, then round the sides. Afterward, use a 4-way foam emery board to rough file, then fine file any snags. Place a few dabs of olive oil on the cuticles, and you're ready to rock your sandals. Keep up with filing every week.

MANICURE/PEDICURE TOOL KIT:

Here are a few basic supplies for your home manicure set-up:
- Cotton balls and cotton swabs
- Non-acetone nail polish remover
- 4-way foam emery board with rough filing, fine filing, smoothing, and buffing
- Orange sticks
- One small and one large nail clipper, plus cuticle scissors
- Top coat and base coat clear polish
- Colored polishes in several shades
- Cuticle nourishing cream (make your own!)
- Exfoliating wand to keep soles of feet smooth

MAKE YOUR OWN HAIR-CARE PRODUCTS

It's a shame that so many of the products we put on our hair are full of chemicals. But be assured that there are healthy alternatives, especially if you are willing to create hair-care products yourself from a few simple ingredients.

NATURAL BEAUTY

It's not only possible to make conditioners and masks to revitalize dank, lusterless hair, but you can also create natural shampoos using essential oils and castile soap, a hard soap made with an olive-oil base and no synthetic detergents. Let your imagination reign as you think up new combinations of essential oils to scent your personalized hair products.

Nature's Own Shampoo: This basic cleanser requires ¼ cup water, ¼ cup pure castile soap, and ½ teaspoon organic soybean or sunflower oil. Mix the ingredients together in a bottle and use like regular shampoo. Try adding a few drops of your favorite essential oil.

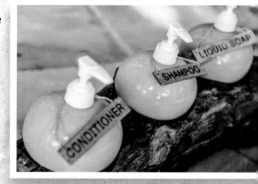

Restoring Shampoo: This recipe hydrates dry hair and adds luster. Combine ¼ cup castile soap, ¼ cup aloe vera gel, 1 teaspoon pure glycerin, and ¼ teaspoon

Shampoo, conditioner, and liquid soap

avocado oil. Store mixture in a bottle and shake well before use. Apply like normal shampoo but let the lather sit for several minutes before rinsing with cool water.

Shampoo for Kids: Make a child-friendly hair cleanser by combining 4 ounces of almond or sunflower oil, 4 tablespoons of baby shampoo, and 10 drops of your child's favorite essential oil. Take a trip to the health-food store and let them decide which oils best fit their personality.

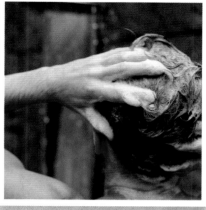
Make your own shampoo

Honey Conditioning Mask: Honey can boost shine and add volume to hair. Mix 1 tablespoon honey with 2 tablespoons coconut oil. Flip your hair over your head and apply from roots to tips. Leave on for 20 minutes then rinse well in a hot shower—all the ingredients should disperse in the heat. You can also prepare this mask with olive oil.

Enriching Hair Mask: Avocado is rich in vitamins and essential fatty acids that are perfect for rehabbing brittle hair. Combine 1 cubed avocado, 2 tablespoons honey, and 1 tablespoon extra-virgin olive oil. Blend the mixture until smooth. Apply to hair and leave on for an hour before rinsing.

Anti-frizz Therapy: Borage oil has a long history of reducing frizz and hydrating dry hair. It can be rubbed into the scalp to moisturize the skin and prevent dandruff. It can also eliminate oxidative stress in the scalp and boost hair growth, even with someone who is beginning to go bald. Test for irritation on a small patch of skin.

DIY: Healthy Hair Spray

No chemicals here, just citrus oils. Chop up ½ orange and ½ lemon and boil the pieces in 2 cups of water until the liquid is reduced by half. Strain and pour into a spray bottle; use a few spritzes to hold hair in place. Will keep in the refrigerator for up to 2 weeks.

Hair Color Helpers: A chamomile tea rinse can enhance the color of blond hair. A rinse of 3 tablespoons apple cider vinegar diluted in a cup of water will bring out red highlights in chestnut hair.

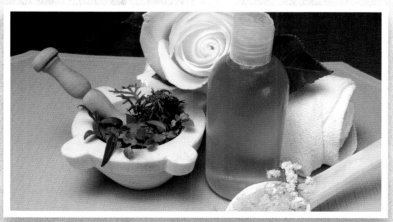
Homemade shampoo

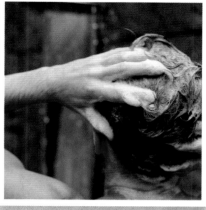

DE-STRESSING TOOLS

One of the mainstays of the spa experience is the hands-on massage. You can help relieve or loosen taut muscles yourself using a variety of tools, including beaded back massagers, electric muscle massagers, and spiky foot massage balls.

At the end of a busy day, most people find they are carrying a lot of tension in the back and shoulders and also experiencing a cramping feeling or pain in the feet. In case you don't have an in-house masseuse or reflexologist to help you find relief, there are tools you can purchase that will get the job done.

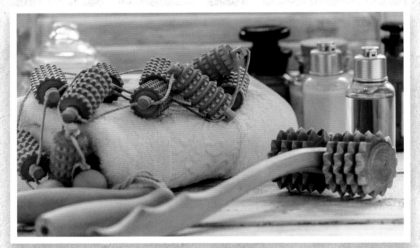

De-stressing Tools

MINI-MASSAGE OPTIONS

In addition to helping to relieve upper-body tension, back massagers make a good pre-exercise step. The current thinking is that before you stretch, perform yoga, or do any sort of gym routine or workout, it helps to warm up your muscles. Back massagers accomplish this by easing away the tightness and stiffness in several muscle groups, allowing you a wider range of motion once you start to move in earnest. They also allow you to focus on certain areas, such as a crick in the neck or a sore shoulder.

Wooden Roller: This simple tool consists of rows of rounded beads strung on corded rope with wooden handles. You swing the beads

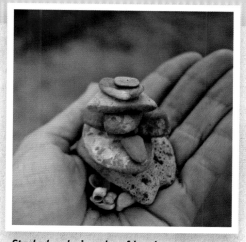

Stacked rocks in palm of hand

behind you and move your arms back and forth, like a cross-country skier, rolling the beads across your neck, back, shoulders, buttocks, and waist. You can really get a good waist swivel going once you master the correct motion, giving yourself an aerobic experience as well. There are also small, handheld wooden rollers that focus on the neck and shoulders.

Electronic Massagers: These devices can be chair cushions (often heated), car seats, or handheld mini-massagers that vibrate or pulse and help ease back pain and tension. The handheld variety is ideal for the home spa—it can be used anywhere on the body there is tension or tightness. Just make sure to keep it away from any water sources.

Foot Massage Ball: This spiky plastic ball that looks like a dog toy is actually a great way to ease your tired feet. You can either sit down and alternately run the bare right and left foot over the ball, or lean one hand on a wall for balance and press the ball beneath one foot, gently shifting it around for a deep massage. Other benefits follow.
• Use the ball to relieve joint pain, strengthen feet and ankles to prevent injury, and assist recovery from a previous injury.
• Rolling your feet over the ball for 15 minutes at bedtime increases circulation, makes you feel calmer, and helps you fall asleep.
• These balls replicate the benefits of reflexology, which has a startling effect on migraine sufferers, who, in studies, more frequently reported relief with foot massage than with the most popular migraine medication.
• Foot massage also helps to address symptoms of anxiety and depression.
• A daily workout with the ball eases the pain of plantar fasciitis and may safely reduce edema in pregnant women.
• Three 10-minute spiky ball sessions a week can lower blood pressure.

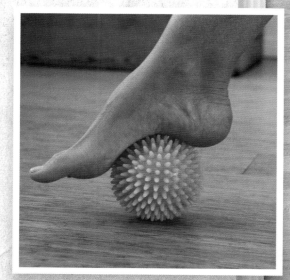

Rubber massage ball

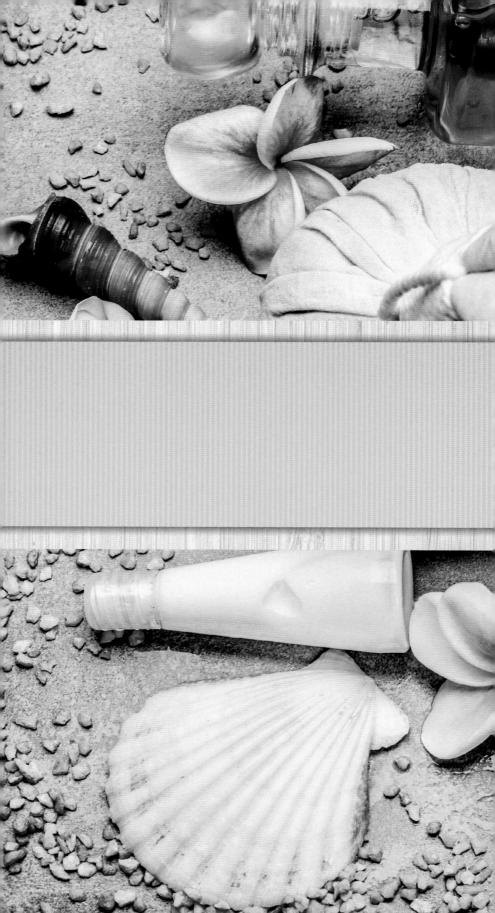

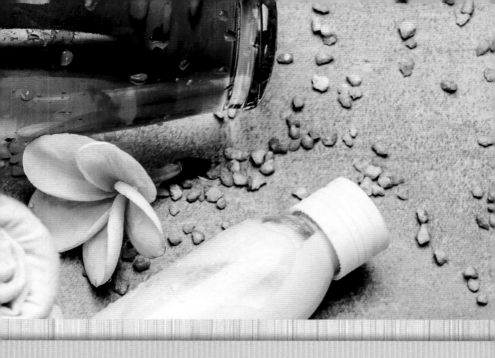

CHAPTER 6

MASSAGE AND TOUCH THERAPIES

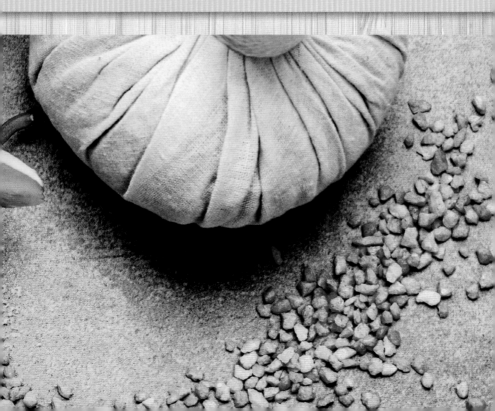

MASSAGE AND TOUCH THERAPIES

A massage can be much more than a once-yearly indulgence at the day spa. It is an ancient practice, which is increasingly being understood to have far-reaching benefits in terms of improving physical and mental health and overall well-being. Incorporating massage into your weekly or monthly wellness routine can also provide an invaluable tool for addressing specific health problems.

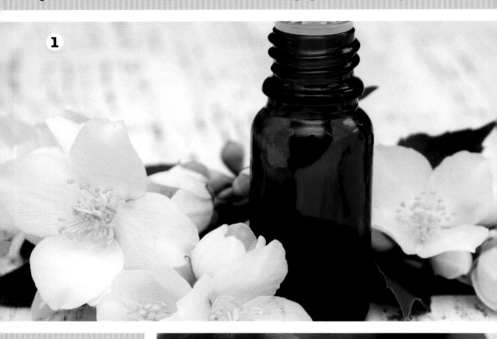

1

1 Massage oil
  with jasmine
  flowers
2 Hot stone
  massage
3 Massage
4 Massage room
  in Shanghai
5 Modern
  wellness center
6 Essential oil
  for ayurveda
  massage

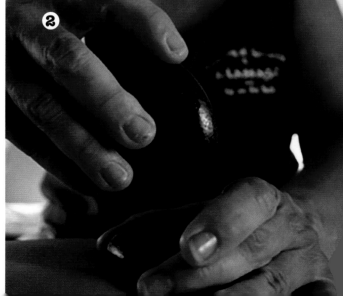

2

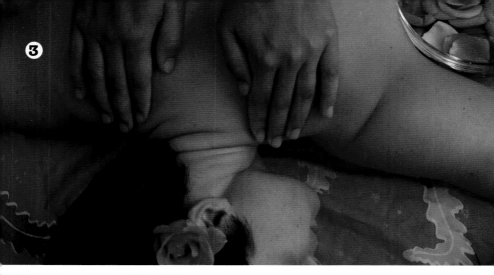

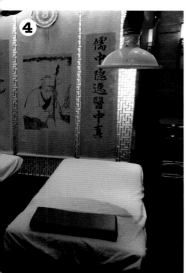

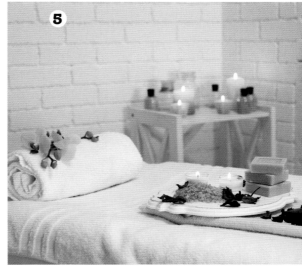

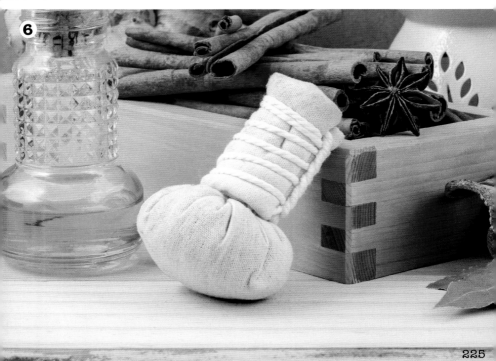

A HISTORY OF MASSAGE

Massage is loosely defined as the targeted pressing, rubbing, and manipulating of soft body tissues—muscles, connective tissue, tendons, and ligaments—with the aim of improving one's physical and mental state, including increased flexibility and range of motion.

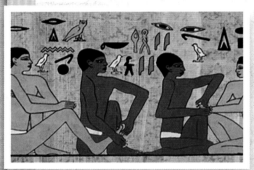

Wall painting found in the tomb of Ankhmahor

There are currently dozens of types of massage schools and methods—called modalities—though they can be broadly categorized into rehabilitative massage and relaxation massage. Modalities such as Swedish massage, reflexology, and acupressure are becoming increasingly accessible at local spas, salons, yoga studios, hotels, and chiropractors, as well as in private physical therapy practices.

Massage therapy originated thousands of years ago, with its earliest testimonials found as far back as ancient China and Egypt. Countless cultures worldwide have practiced and developed their own forms of massage, which have been handed down from generation to generation. It is considered to be one of the world's oldest forms of "healing art."

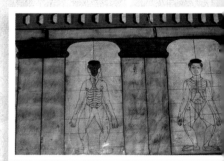

Ancient thai massage pressure points on wall of buddhist temple in Thailand

Yet today, although many people treat themselves to the occasional massage as a birthday treat or vacation indulgence, few know the ancient roots and thousand-year history of massage worldwide. It is not surprising, however that healing touch is such a ubiquitous practice of humans everywhere. Touch is so much a part of our relationship to our bodies and to one another. As soon as societies began to form and develop, social touch too developed into what we today call massage.

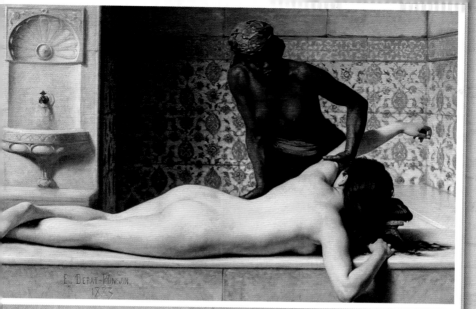

Massage at the Hammam, 1883

TWO SCHOOLS OF MASSAGE

Recently it has become easier than ever to find a range of massage alternatives, even at your local spa. All of these options can be overwhelming if you're a newcomer to the world of modern inter-disciplinary massage. Most types of massage can be categorized into Eastern-based and Western-based approaches. Both types are effective, so it all depends on what you're hoping to accomplish from your massage.

Eastern Massage: Massage techniques developed in the East tend to take a holistic approach to healing, based on balance and energy flow within the body, mind, and spirit. There is a common belief that stimulating certain pressure points and soothing others can promote the flow of energy as it travels around the body along certain interconnected pathways. If you have persistent knee pain, for example, a Chinese massage practitioner may look at your tongue or focus on points on your wrist as a means to understanding the state of your immune system, rather than look at your knee itself.

Western Massage: Massage as a way to increase general well-being has only taken hold in Western culture relatively recently. In general, Western-based massage methods tend to be more focused and diagnostic in nature. They emphasize targeting specific trouble or tightness in the muscles and treating it through practiced touch therapy. Yet there is always an element of relaxation and mind-body peace involved as well.

If you're confused about which method of massage to try, talk to a massage professional about your specific goals and concerns. There are a lot of options out there, and massage is not one size fits all. It's about finding what works best for you.

SWEDISH MASSAGE

Swedish massage is the most widespread type of massage in Western culture—it's likely the modality you see advertised in your local spas and salons. If you've ever wondered what this popular Scandinavian massage therapy entails, look no further.

Swedish massage, often called a "classical" massage, offers a number of different techniques combined into one session. Its aim is to promote the general health and well-being of the recipient, while

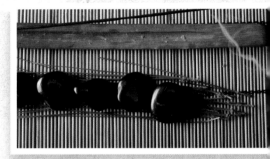

Volcanic hot-stones

increasing the level of relaxation in the entire body. As a healing treatment it attempts to energize the body by stimulating circulation and promoting looseness in the targeted muscles. It incorporates five basic strokes that circle around the heart and manipulate the soft

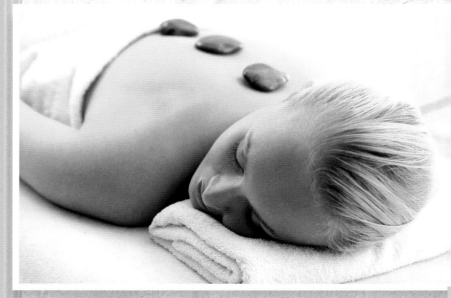

Hot stone massage

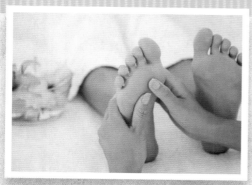

Foot massage

body tissue in different ways. Your masseuse will use a combination of gliding, kneading, rubbing, vibration, and percussive and tapping motions to target specific muscles. Above all, it is a "soothing" massage, rather than a high-pressure massage.

First developed in Sweden by Per Henrik Ling in the mid-nineteenth century, the method combined his background in gymnastics with his know of physiology and of Chinese, Egyptian, Greek, and Roman techniques. Ling introduced the modality to the United States in 1858 as the "Swedish movement cure." It is typically applied as a full-body massage that can be slow and gentle or rigorous.

BENEFITS OF SWEDISH MASSAGE

There are many reasons to give Swedish massage a try. Whether you're feeling stiff and achy or you're just looking for some well-earned relaxation, this can be a great way to find relief for what ails you.

Not only will Swedish massage loosen your muscles and make you more flexible, it is also known to have other major health benefits, including raising your "good" hormone levels, improving sleep, boosting your immune system, fighting off headaches and migraines, and generally making you feel better. Swedish massage is the perfect antidote to a busy life.

A VERSATILE TECHNIQUE: Swedish massage can provide the following healing benefits.
- Pain management
- Increased blood flow
- Increased flexibility
- Reduced stress
- Improved immune system
- Elimination of waste products
- Enhanced sleep quality
- Relief of tension-related headaches
- Greater energy
- Elevated mood

WHAT TO EXPECT

At the start of the massage session, you will be asked to undress and provided with a towel. If you are uncomfortable with this, it's okay to keep your underwear on. Your masseuse will tell you to lie face down or face up on the table. The masseuse begins by applying a lubricating oil or lotion. As the massage starts, let your masseuse know if there are any specific points that you want him or her to target or if you begin to experience pain. You will likely begin facing down and the masseuse will work up from your feet. Once you turn face up, the session will typically end with a facial massage. A thorough Swedish massage should take an average of 75 minutes.

SWEDISH MASSAGE TECHNIQUES

Swedish massage is known for the development and deployment of a number of basic hands-on movements that facilitate the release of energy and the soothing of tense muscles. These are applied in five steps: effleurage, pettrisage, tapotement, friction, and vibration.

ALL THE RIGHT MOVES

In both Western- and Eastern-style massage, the goal is to mobilize the body's own healing properties, but with Western-style massage the focus is more on muscles, ligaments, tendons, connective tissues, and the cardiovascular system. This resulted in the development of a variety of gliding, kneading, and percussive strokes along with deep, circular movements and vibrations.

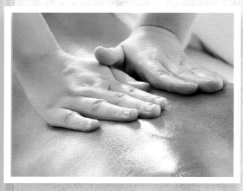

Effleurage

Effleurage: Effleurage consists of stroking or gliding movements. Stroking movements start and finish a massage session as the masseuse works into or out of deeper, more intense movements. These movements are applied with the entire palm surface of the hand, starting with superficial strokes to apply the oil or cream. Using light, superficial pressure, the direction of the strokes is typically applied toward the heart or away from heart.

Pettrisage: Petrissage consists of compression movements. These include kneading, skin rolling, wringing, and frictions created with finger or thumb. Petrissage movements are performed with intermittent pressure either with

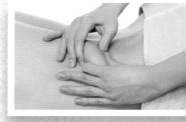

Lower-back petrissage

one or both hands. The pressure is firmly and smoothly applied, then relaxed. The movement is then shifted to the next adjacent area and repeated. The degree of pressure exerted must be reduced on less muscular areas.

Tapotement: Tapotement movements include beating, pounding, cupping, hacking, and frictions. All these movements are stimulating and should only be used if a general toning effect is required from the massage rather than relaxation.

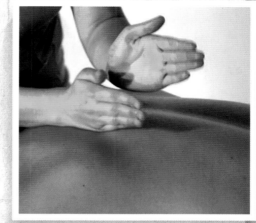

Tapotement

Friction: Frictions are concentrated movements using focused pressure on a small area of the surface tissues, moving them over the underlying bone structures. The movement completes several small circles over a limited area, placing a degree of stretch in the muscles; pressure is then relaxed and the hand moves on to the next area without losing contact.

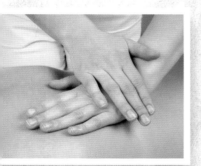

Vibration massage

Vibrations: Vibration and shaking movements produce a tremor in the tissues, but they are very different in their uses. Vibration is a single or double-handed technique that applies a fine shaking or tremor to the area by hand or fingertips. Vibrations include thumb vibrations and finger vibrations. They are fine trembling movements performed on or along the nerve path by the fingers or the thumb. The shaking method is similar to the above but with a rhythmic shaking movement or tremor applied.

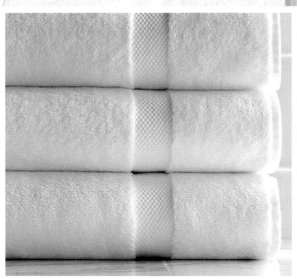

PRESSURE POINT MASSAGE

Long before the existence of European massage techniques, Asian cultures had pioneered a form of massage based on the body's pressure points. It is still one of the best ways to relieve muscular pain and discomfort.

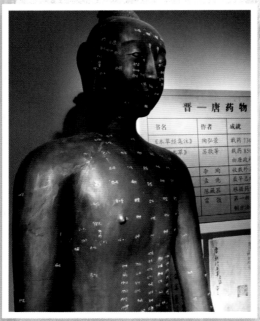

The Bronze Man, used in bygone times to display pressure points

Pressure point massage focuses on certain key points in the body where tightness and stiffness tend to accumulate. Anyone who spends long hours at the office recognizes the feeling of pressure or tension building up after sitting hunched at their desk all day. Instead of relying on over-the-counter pain relief, pressure point massage can be a great antidote to this daily discomfort.

WHAT ARE PRESSURE POINTS?

Pressure points, also known as meridians in Chinese medicine, are specific points of the body where energy tends to build up. By incorporating a type of massage that targets these pressure points, your masseuse can open up the surrounding blood vessels so that your energy, or chi, can flow more freely.

WHAT IS PRESSURE POINT MASSAGE?

Suppose that after hours sitting at the computer, you begin feeling a deep, sharp pain somewhere beside your shoulder blade. Without even thinking, you reach back to the point of pain and attempt to massage it. This, in essence, is a rudimentary form of pressure point massage. While this form of self-administered massage can be helpful,

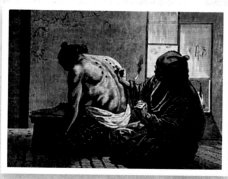
Historic image depicting accupuncture

approaching a more practiced pressure point massage specialist might be the best way to find the relief you need. There are several types and techniques of pressure point massage. They all aim, however, to concentrate on certain pressure points in order to relieve different ailments and pain affecting the body. The most important thing to remember is that your pain does not always correlate to a pressure point in the same part of the body. This is why you should leave it to the experts.

TYPES OF PRESSURE POINT MASSAGE

By stimulating certain pressure points and nerve centers, a masseuse can alleviate all kinds of health problems. Types of pressure point massage include shiatsu, acupressure, and reflexology. Once you learn more about each one, you can find the type that is best for you.

Shiatsu Massage: This word literally translates in Japanese to "finger pressure," which gives you some insight into how this technique works. During a shiatsu session, the practitioner will use his or her fingers, thumbs, and palms to put pressure on specific points on the body, depending on the patient's needs. Some shiatsu massages concentrate only on pressure points, while other practitioners incorporate more general body and energy work into the session. Styles include Zen, macrobiotic, healing, Namikoshi, movement, and Hara.

DIY: Ease Shoulder Pain

Neck and shoulder pain are often the result of stress or prolonged poor posture and can lead to tension headaches. Specialists suggest using several pressure points for the relief of shoulder pain, including this most commonly used technique.
• Spread the fingers of one hand wide apart, and with your other hand grab hold of the web of stretched skin between your thumb and pointer finger.
• Apply a firm pressure until you feel a light ache.
• Hold for five seconds.
• Release and repeat three more times.

Acupressure Massage: Acupressure has its earliest roots in traditional Chinese medicine, which has incorporated this practice for the past 2,000 years. Much like acupuncture, which uses tiny needles to stimulate certain key pressure points, in acupressure massage your masseuse will apply finger-pressure at certain meridians, or pressure points. If you're squeamish about being stuck with many tiny needles, give acupressure massage a try instead.

REFLEXOLOGY

Many people are under the misconception that reflexology is just a fancy word for a foot massage. What this modality incorporates are centuries-old methods that use the feet as conduits for healing other parts of the body.

A reflexology session may feel similar to a foot massage, in that a practitioner will focus on manually rubbing and massaging your feet. The aim of a foot massage, however, is to provide relief from any discomfort in the muscles of the feet. Reflexology, on the other hand, aims to use the feet as a portal to improve well-being in the rest of the body. Underlying this practice is the belief that the feet can be mapped out into an atlas of "zones," each of which can alter another zone in the body.

Reflexologists believe that these reflex points in the feet and hands correspond to different body organs and systems, and that stimulating them can create real benefits for the person's health. For example, reflexology holds that a specific spot in the arch of the foot corresponds to the bladder. When a reflexologist uses their thumbs or fingers to apply appropriate pressure to this area, it may affect bladder functioning.

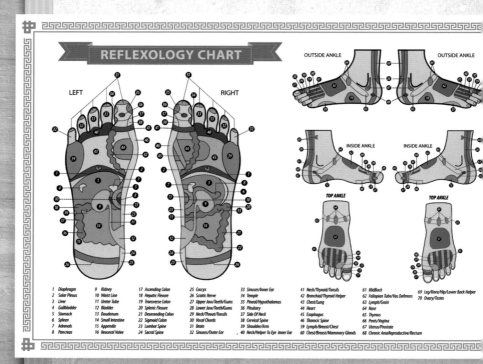

Foot and hand reflexology chart

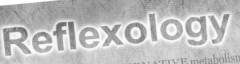

Reflexology banner

In addition to manipulating the pressure points on the foot, reflexologists sometimes work on the hands or ears to trigger healing and relaxation as well.

A BRIEF HISTORY

There are records that some form of hand and foot therapy began in China around 2330 BC and, according to tomb depictions, also in Egypt at about the same time. As the centuries passed, these practices undoubtedly spread to much of the civilized world. In 1582, Dr. Adamus and Dr. A'tatis published a European volume on an integral element of reflexology called zone

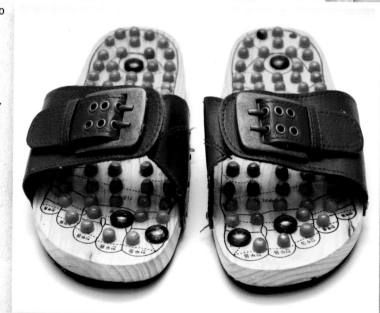

Foot reflexology shoes

therapy. American physician William H. Fitzgerald—frequently called the father of reflexology—theorized on what he called zone analgesia and in 1917 described ten vertical zones that extended the length of the body. Fitzgerald had learned that applying pressure to these zones not only relieved pain, it often eliminated the underlying causes as well. Dr. Shelby Riley, who worked closely with Dr. Fitzgerald, added horizontal zones across the hands and feet.

REFLEXOLOGY

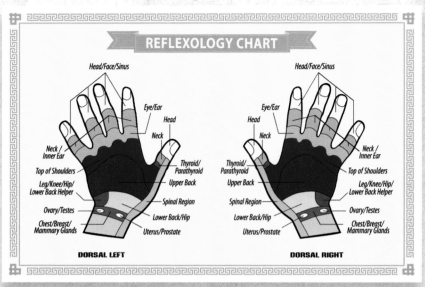

REFLEXOLOGY CHART

Head/Face/Sinus

Eye/Ear

Head

Neck

Neck / Inner Ear

Top of Shoulders

Leg/Knee/Hip/ Lower Back Helper

Ovary/Testes

Chest/Breast/ Mammary Glands

Thyroid/ Parathyroid

Upper Back

Spinal Region

Lower Back/Hip

Uterus/Prostate

DORSAL LEFT

Head/Face/Sinus

Eye/Ear

Head

Neck

Thyroid/ Parathyroid

Upper Back

Spinal Region

Lower Back/Hip

Uterus/Prostate

Neck / Inner Ear

Top of Shoulders

Leg/Knee/Hip/ Lower Back Helper

Ovary/Testes

Chest/Breast/ Mammary Glands

DORSAL RIGHT

Reflexology hand chart

Zone therapy was modified in the 1930s and 1940s by American nurse and physiotherapist Eunice D. Ingham. She maintained that the feet and hands were especially sensitive, and mapped the entire body into "reflexes" on the feet, calling her new method reflexology. Her book, *Stories the Feet Can Tell Thru Reflexology*, was published in seven languages and spread reflexology well beyond the United States.

BENEFITS OF REFLEXOLOGY

No one will argue that a foot massage feels really, really good. But

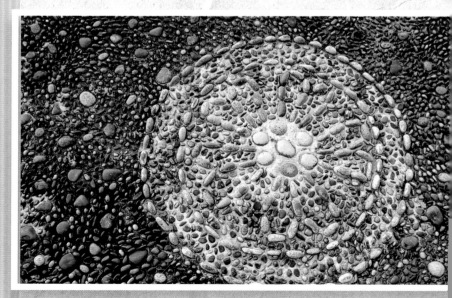

Close-up on pebble stones at foot reflexology park

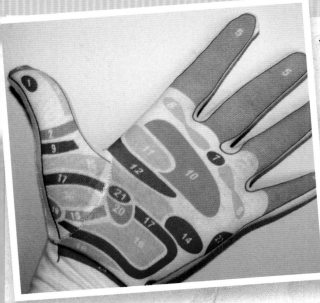

Reflexology glove

treating yourself to a reflexology session can go far beyond the pleasurable effects of a foot rub. The practice and purpose of reflexology goes deeper than easing tired muscles. It can be used to address anything from headaches to sinus problems to bladder infections. If sensitivity or tenderness is felt when certain parts of the foot are stimulated, it usually indicates bodily weakness or imbalance in the corresponding organ. Your reflexologist can then apply repeated pressure and manipulate the nerve endings of the foot to help clear any channels of blocked energy and ultimately improve overall health and balance.

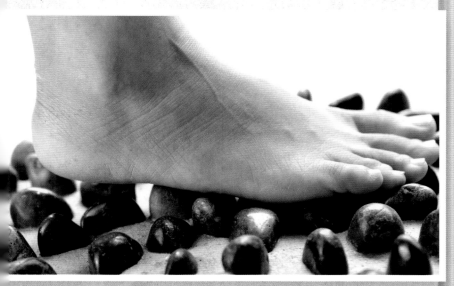

Reflexology path

WHAT DOES IT DO?

Although reflexology on its own cannot be used to diagnose or cure diseases, millions of people around the world use it as a complementary treatment for conditions such as anxiety, asthma, cancer treatment, cardiovascular issues, diabetes, headaches, kidney function, PMS, and sinusitis. It is also believed to boost the immune system and improve overall well-being.

DEEP TISSUE MASSAGE

Keeping up with the ever-increasing demands of modern life can take its toll on body and mind. For persistent aches and muscle tightness, a deep tissue massage might be just what the holistic doctor ordered.

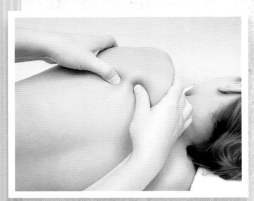
Shoulder massage

Constant stress, deadlines, workplace drama, and other daily frustrations don't just pass through us without doing harm. These experiences can accumulate stress in our bodies, causing a buildup of muscle tension that may exacerbate or even cause physical injury. When even a Swedish massage doesn't bring relief, it might be time to go deeper.

TARGETING DEEP TISSUES
Though some of the strokes used in deep tissue massage feel similar to Swedish massage, this technique is intended to target the much deeper layer of connective tissue and muscle throughout the body. Using slow strokes to apply pressure, the massage focuses on areas of preexisting pain and tension.

Injuries or chronic muscle tension can create adhesions, or knots, which form in the tendons, ligaments, and muscles. These knots will feel rigid and painful, and can block blood circulation, hinder range of motion, and cause inflammation and pain. When the muscles are deeply massaged, blood flow throughout the body increases, reducing inflammation and relieving pain. Repeated sessions can break up and even eliminate the presence of scar tissue surrounding the muscle.

BENEFITS OF DEEP MUSCLE MASSAGE
Deep tissue massage usually focuses on a specific problem, such as chronic muscle pain or injury rehabilitation and can provide relief from the following complaints:
• Low back pain

- Upper neck or back pain
- Limited mobility
- Recovery from injuries (whiplash, falls)
- Repetitive strain injuries (carpal tunnel syndrome)
- Postural problems
- Muscle tension in the legs, buttocks, and lower back
- Osteoarthritic pain and sciatica
- Sports concerns of athletes; tennis elbow
- Piriformis syndrome
- Fibromyalgia

WHAT TO EXPECT

At the beginning of the massage, oil or lotion is applied and then lighter pressure is used to warm up and prep the muscles. Then you will begin to receive stimulation in the deep muscle and connective tissue from the therapist's hands, elbows, forearms, fingertips, and/or knuckles in order to relieve the tense trouble spots in your body. You will be asked to relax and breathe deeply during this time, allowing your body to release tension and heal. The two main techniques used are known as stripping—deep, gliding pressure along the length of the muscle fibers using the elbow, forearm, knuckles, and thumbs—and friction, pressure applied across the grain of a muscle to release adhesions and realign tissue fibers.

At certain points during the massage, you may feel discomfort or even pain as the massage therapist works on areas where you have deep knots or a buildup of scar tissue. You should always let the masseuse know when you're feeling pain, so he or she can adjust their technique or further prep tense muscles. Pain isn't necessarily good, and it shouldn't be taken as a sign that the massage is working. Your body will typically tense up in response to pain, making it harder for the therapist to reach deep muscles. Some stiffness and soreness for a day or two following the massage is normal.

WHAT IS ROLFING?

Unlike massage, which focuses on relaxation and relief of muscle discomfort, the goal of rolfing—also known as structural integration—is improving body alignment and functioning. These goals are achieved through tissue manipulation and myofascial release. The modality is named for its creator, American biochemist Dr. Ida P. Rolf, and its benefits include improved athletic ability, relief for TMJ and chronic back pain, improved posture and spine health, and improved asthma and breathing in general.

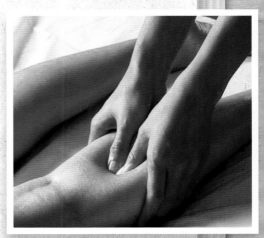

Calf massage

ALTERNATIVE THERAPIES

You probably consider yourself open-minded—wellness and well-being appeals to you and you've tried yoga and drink kombucha. But maybe you're still a skeptic about the pseudo-spiritual realm of alternative medicine and energy healing.

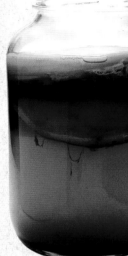

Kombucha

There's no shortage of advice and testimonials pertaining to holistic health these days. Yet, many people still question the legitimacy and effectiveness of alternative medicines and therapies. Massage, however, is not merely a new age fringe form of spiritual healing—many alternative massage therapies that are popular today have been tried and tested for thousands of years. In addition to the physical benefits, many alternative healing methods also address mental, spiritual, psychological, and emotional factors that might be triggering pain and discomfort.

TYPES OF ALTERNATIVE THERAPIES

While there many types of alternative massage therapies, a handful have emerged into mainstream practice. A number offer ways to recondition your everyday behaviors, the ones that caused the buildup of stress and tightness in the muscles in the first place.

Alexander Technique: Alexander Technique is aimed at changing habits of movement and posture in ways that promote better physical health and reduce problems. Many of us develop bad postural habits in how we sit, stand, and walk. These habits then contribute to persistent physical problems, such as back, neck, and shoulder pain; restricted movement; and general tiredness. Alexander Technique helps individuals to understand the correct movements and postures, and subsequently learn to break their bad habits.

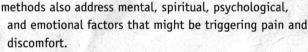

Movement Awareness: Studies in basic body and movement awareness have found an increase in people who suffer from a lack of realization of their physical body, emotions, and spacial boundaries as they relate to others and to their physical surroundings. This then affects their quality of movement, daily functions, habits, and health. Movement awareness therapy aims to reestablish new ways of being and an awareness of the body through targeted therapy.

Tension Release Therapy: Many people who seek out tension relief therapy experience chronic muscle tension due to stress or chronic use of certain muscles. Tension release therapy, essentially, is another form of massage, but one practiced by a physician, chiropractor, or occupational therapist, rather than in a massage parlor. The specialist will follow a similar pattern of manual muscle work, stimulating the tight tissue layer by layer.

Rosen Method Therapy: Rosen Method Therapy is different than other forms of massage or bodywork. It is characterized by gentle, directive touch. Using hands that listen to, rather than manipulate the body, the practitioner focuses on areas of chronic muscle tension as well as slowly releasing unconscious feelings, attitudes, and memories surrounding the body. The aim of this practice is psychosomatic, meaning it uses the mind as a tool to affect the body and vice versa.

Trager Work: Trager Approach is based on the premise that discomfort, pain, and reduced function are physical symptoms of accumulated tension that result from accidents, weak posture, fear, emotional blockages, and daily stress. It focuses on reducing these unnatural patterns of movement and eliminating neuromuscular tension by using gentle, rhythmic rocking motions. These rhythmic movements can create a state of deep relaxation, which therapists say can allow the body and mind to achieve a state of balance and integration.

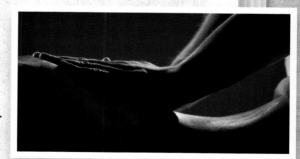

Trager therapy

Bioenergetics: Bioenergetics is another form of psychosomatic treatment that emphasizes the connection between body and mind. This approach posits that the psychological defenses an individual uses to cope with stress or pain manifest themselves in the physical body in unique muscular patterns that may inhibit self-expression. Treatment sessions attempt to illuminate old, ineffective patterns of constrictive movement, and then teach the client new ones.

FINDING A PROFESSIONAL MASSEUSE

So, you're inspired by what you've read. Your fingers are already itching to google "massage therapist near me." Great! Here's what you should know now that you're ready to begin looking for a professional masseuse.

Before searching for a professional, ask yourself "What am I looking for?" Are you an athlete with performance issues or someone recovering from an injury? Do you experience chronic muscle tightness and discomfort? Or maybe you're just looking for some much-needed relaxation and energy renewal. There are many options for bodywork, massage, movement therapy, and energy work therapy, so it's important to do your research. Knowing what you hope to achieve will help you pinpoint the types of treatments that will help you the most and which specialists offer those treatments.

Professional masseuse massaging shoulder

FINDING A SPECIALIST

When entrusting your well-being to a virtual stranger, it is extremely important to find a specialist who is knowledgeable, trained, and certified in the type of work they are providing. No matter what modality you decide on, make sure the specialist in question has received the proper certification.

Personal referrals are a good place to start. If a friend has been raving about her new massage miracle worker, ask for the person's contact info. Get the specialist on the phone, explain what you're looking for, and ask if you would benefit from the specific treatment he or she provides. Even if that person is not the best fit, he or she can likely refer you to someone else who is. Or consider an online directory:

"Massagetique" and other similar directories list professionals whose backgrounds and credentials have already been verified and approved.

WHAT TO ASK YOUR THERAPIST

Once you have a therapist in mind, there are several key questions you need to ask before scheduling an appointment.

Background: Ask the therapist how long he or she has been a massage therapist and what kind of training he or she has. Ask which style of massage he or she specializes in and where else he or she has practiced. Make sure the therapist is comfortable working with your specific needs or health condition. (Once you visit your new masseuse, that person should do an intake interview with his or her own set of questions.)

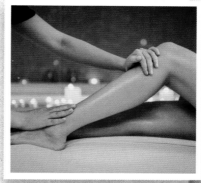

Woman lying on massage table

Policies: You will want to know how far in advance you need to book your massage and what the cancellation policy is. Do you need to bring certain clothes, for example a bathing suit, gym shorts, or workout bra, to wear during the massage? Does the specialist need to see a prescription from a physician or an exercise plan from a physical therapist? You will also want to call your health-care provider to see if your sessions are covered. Many are.

Pricing: Pricing boards with long lists of services and prices can be intimidating to the uninitiated. Don't be daunted by all the options and add-ons. Before you go to the massage parlor, make the appointment based on exactly what you're looking for. Find out what length sessions are available and what the cost is for each session. Ask if there are different fees for different techniques. Will there be any additional fees or taxes? Do they offer any special rates or discounts? Go in knowing exactly what you want and which service you will be using, and how much you expect to pay.

TIPPING GUIDELINES?

To tip or not to tip can be a touchy subject. Knowing the protocol and expectations beforehand can alleviate a lot of stress and help you enjoy your massage. If you're going to tip, the usual rate is 15–20 percent. It is always appropriate to tip at a spa, on a cruise ship, or in a massage chain. If you are seeing a medical massage therapist or the owner of a medical practice, it is not appropriate to tip.

PERFORMING MASSAGE AT HOME

If having a massage is such an important part of living a healthful lifestyle, why don't we all do it more often? Making regular visits to a spa or massage therapist costs money and takes time . . . but there's always the option of a DIY massage at home.

There's no doubt that getting a massage is good for you, body and mind, but if you have too much going on in your life to plan in a massage each week, consider these options for relieving muscles aches and tension in the comfort of your own home. It's not difficult to ease some cases of muscle imbalance and tightness yourself until you have time to get back to your pro.

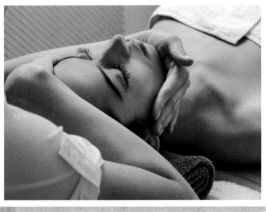
Head and neck massage

DIY MASSAGE TECHNIQUES
There are many self-care techniques you can try to relax or sooth aching muscles. Thankfully, you really don't need lots of expensive equipment or long periods of time. Whenever you're feeling sore, give your body a little TLC with these mini self-massages.

Head/Scalp: This is one of those rare self-massages that you can do pretty much anywhere and at any time to provide a little relaxation and clarity to your body and mind. Place the heels of your palms beneath your hairline on either side of your head, near your temples. Supply pressure inward and upward on your scalp, pulling toward the ceiling on either side. Hold for several seconds and then release. Work in sections across your entire scalp, pulling upward, downward, and side to side.

Face: A self-administered face massage is especially fruitful at the early onset of a headache or migraine. Touch both sets of fingertips to your forehead, where it meets either corner of your hairline. Use your fingertips to press light circles along your hairline and cheekbones,

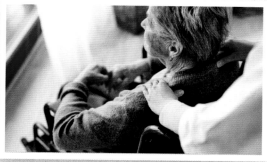

The elderly can greatly benefit from massage too

above your eyebrows, and where your jaw connects. Gently rub your ears and earlobes between your fingertips.

Hands/Forearms: Too much typing and texting? Here's a cure. Relax one arm, palm up, on top of your thigh. Push the heel of your other palm slowly along the forearm toward your wrist. Use enough pressure to feel some heat, but not to give yourself a brush burn. Do the same thing across your open palm all the way down toward your fingertips, and again over the mound of your thumb. Repeat a few times, and switch hands.

Neck/Shoulders: Slouching forward or sitting still for prolonged periods can make shoulder and neck muscles tight. To alleviate this pain at the end of the workday, drop your shoulders so they're not hunched, and slowly tuck your chin to your chest to stretch your neck. Place two or three fingertips on the back of your neck where neck and shoulders meet. Press firmly and hold, releasing when the muscle feels more relaxed. Roll your shoulders forward and back slowly. Repeat as needed.

Lower Back: Place a tennis ball on the floor and lie on it, or position it between your back and the wall. Move your body slowly up and down and side to side so that the ball massages any areas of muscle tightness (avoid your spine to prevent injury). Press hard enough to squish the ball a little but

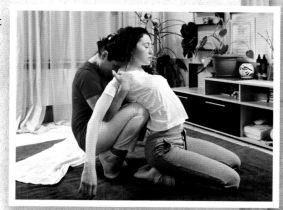

Massage therapist treating patient at home

not so much that it hurts. Just a few minutes of rolling should be sufficient—you don't want to aggravate already irritated tissues.

Thigh: Loosen up tight quads after sitting all day by rolling a tennis ball or foam roller on top of your thighs. You also can use the palm of your hands to make small circles, working your way up the thigh from the knee. Or lean forward and run your elbow in a single stroke along the thigh from the knee toward the torso. Make several passes at slightly different angles along the thigh.

SETTING UP A MASSAGE AREA

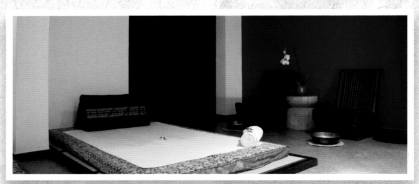

Room for relaxation and massage

One way to incorporate massage into your daily life is to prepare a dedicated space in which to perform it, in part of your bedroom, say, or in a corner of a finished basement.

A dedicated massage area not only allows you to perform mini-massages on yourself, but it also means you can offer body massages to your spouse or significant other, and he or she can then return the favor. Setting plays a huge part in creating a relaxing and therapeutic massage area. Bright lights, intrusive noises, or clutter may make you unable to relax and enjoy the experience.

MAXIMIZE YOUR SPACE

One important rule of setting up a restorative massage space is making sure you have whatever you need at your fingertips. This doesn't mean filling up every corner of the room with supplies, however—it's just the opposite. The space needs to be efficient as well as relaxing.

Clear Out: Filter out unneeded items—to lessen the amount of clutter, keep only what you need to perform basic massage techniques.

Organize your tools: Keep all your supplies and equipment neatly stored away but handy. Fabric bins or baskets set on a low shelf get the job done and look attractive.

Keep a wide space around the table: Position your massage table, supplies, and any other furniture in such a way that you have plenty of room to walk around freely.

SET THE MOOD

Nothing ruins a good massage quicker than irksome background distractions. Even small disturbances such as the sound of a distant TV can kill the relaxing mood. Pay attention to ambiance if you want the optimal amount of tranquility.

Light: Light the room with a few low-wattage table lamps or floor spots, or use the light from a window filtered through mini-blinds. Avoid fluorescent lights overhead—they give off significant amounts of blue-spectrum light that can impact relaxation and sleep patterns.

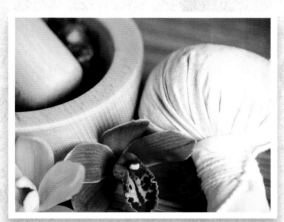

Herbs and massage compress

Noise: Activity from beyond the room or ambient background noises such as traffic, kids playing, or even appliances can also be distracting. Use relaxing music to obscure outside noises.

BUYING A TABLE

You should be able to find a decent massage table for between $100 and $250. Unless you are planning to open a massage practice, this level of comfort and dependability should be fine for you and your family. The two main requirements are that the table be sturdy enough to bear the weight of an adult—and the weight of another adult who is exerting pressure on the first adult—without wobbling, and wide enough for an adult to lie comfortably. To be sure of the width you need, measure the tables at your own massage salon. If you find the table is not well cushioned, you can add extra padding from a thin foam mattress or extra layers of sheets or towels. The area near the face is also crucial—make sure you have a comfortable face cradle or pillow. Place the table on a rug or carpeting so that it does not move around.

WHAT ELSE YOU NEED

If you treat this space like a professional massage salon, you'll need at least a few of the following items.

- Pillows, linens, and towels
- Tissues and wipes
- Lotions and oils of your preference
- A source for your favorite healing scents
- A device to produce soft, ambient music
- A small table or rolling cart to hold supplies

THE BEST IT CAN BE

Massage, ideally, should be a source of relaxation, comfort, and relief. But like any health or beauty appointment, you may find that just getting to the parlor or salon on time can be stressful—hardly the outcome you want.

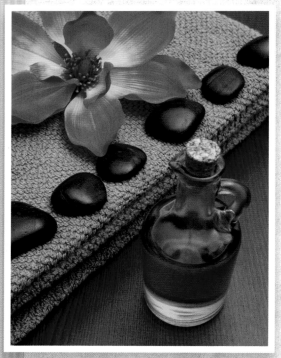

Massage oil with massage stones

Your massage appointment should not make your existing problems worse or create undue stress for you. Here are some tips for getting the most out of your massage, as well as certain troublemakers you'll want to avoid.

Don't be in a rush! Never hurry to and from your massage appointments. Nothing ruins a massage faster than running in the door late, your adrenaline pumping, stressed to the max, and muscles tightened up. Or, conversely, worrying throughout the session about finishing exactly on time because you have to race out the door to your next errand or to work. Instead, schedule your massage for when you have plenty of time on either side of the session, so you can arrive early and unrushed

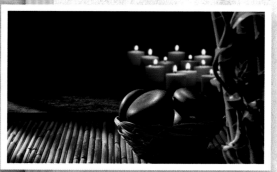

Soothing atmosphere of a wellness holistic spa

and leave in a similar state. You want to carry the calm created during your visit as far as you can throughout the day . . . and hopefully longer.

Alcohol: Restrict your alcohol intake before having a massage. Massage stimulates nearly all the systems in the body, and if you have been drinking, you can wind up feeling really lousy during and after your massage. If possible, avoid alcohol altogether the day you receive a massage, or limit yourself to a glass of wine or a single beer.

Caffeine: Do not drink an excessive amount of caffeinated beverages before a session. If you're a coffee or soda fan, stop drinking them at least 6–8 hours before your massage appointment. The body can achieve a deeper state of relaxation during your massage if your nervous system is not jacked up on caffeine.

Unhealthy Foods: Don't eat fast food or junk food before or after your massage. It's never a good idea to chow down a deluxe cheeseburger and fries just before receiving a massage. After a hefty salt- and fat-laden meal, you'll feel lethargic, bloated, and uncomfortably full. Massage tends to heighten or deepen our ability to feel and sense, so feed your body healthy, nutrient-rich foods before and after to get the most out of your treatment. Your body will thank you

WHEN TO AVOID A MASSAGE:

Even though a massage might always sound like a good idea, if certain medical situations arise then its probably best to stay home and treat your medical condition first. Then, when you're feeling fit again, simply reschedule your appointment. If there are any lingering physical aftereffects of your illness or injury, let your masseuse know.

You should cancel your appointment if you are experiencing any of following:

• You're running a fever or have an elevated temperature.

• You were recently involved in a car accident, sports accident, or fall of some kind.

• You are feeling light-headed, dizzy, or nauseous.

• You are bruised, or have an open wound, rash, or sunburn.

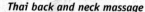

Thai back and neck massage

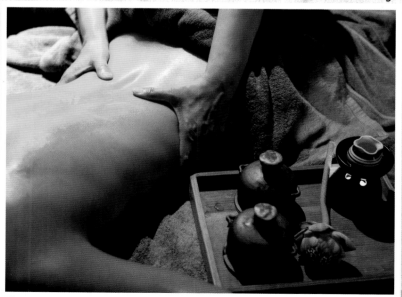

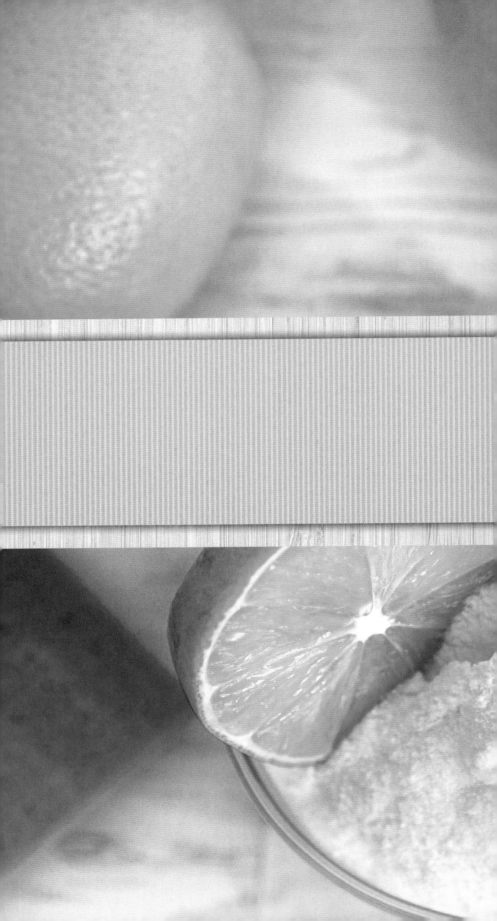

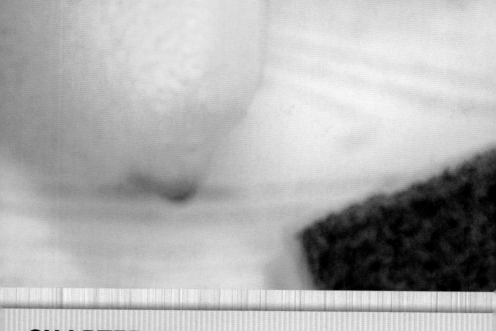

CHAPTER 7

THE NATURALLY HEALTHY HOME

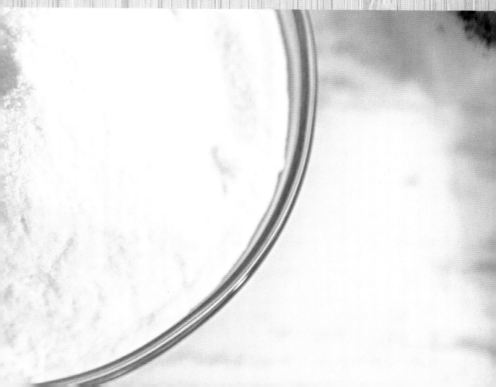

THE NATURALLY HEALTHY HOME

You'd probably be surprised at how many of the products you use every day to clean and disinfect your home or to clear the air pose genuine health risks. Fortunately, Mother Nature has supplied us with numerous safe, healthy cleaners, disinfectants, and air fresheners that you can prepare yourself from items in your pantry.

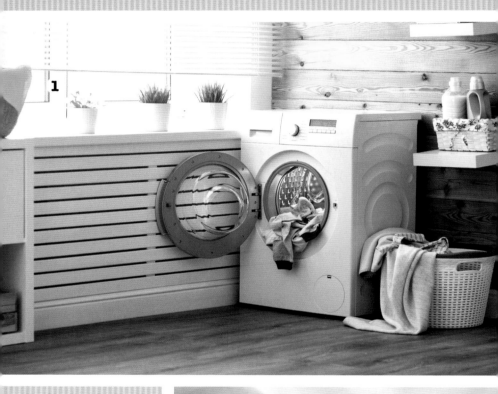

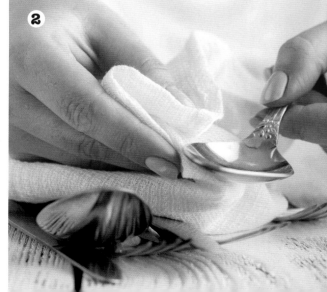

1 Everyday household products can act as a natural way to keep your home sparkling clean
2 Leave your shoes outside if you have small children
3 Baking soda acts as a great product for cleaning silverware
4 Use baking soda for cleaning surfaces

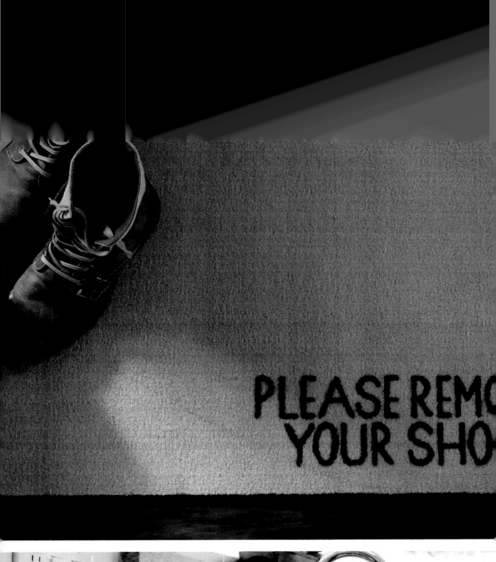

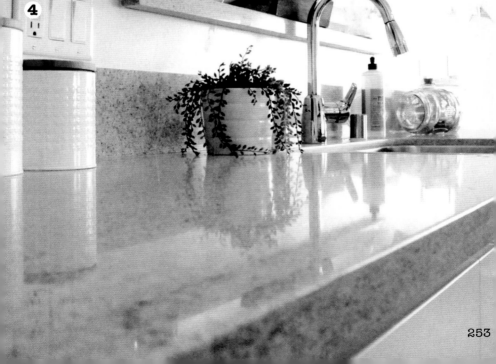

WELCOME TO YOUR HEALTHY HOME

Wellness isn't just about what we put into our bodies or sticking to an exercise plan; it's also about making sure our homes are free of chemical toxins and remaining vigilant about keeping them that way.

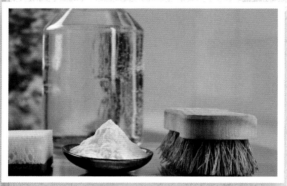

Baking soda makes for an effective cleaner

People in the modern world take the advances of technology for granted. And that includes the host of home cleaners the chemical industry has provided. We think nothing of using four or five different cleaning products—counter wipes; disinfectants; floor, tub, and tile cleaners; spot removers; degreasers—in the course of a day. But what many of us don't realize is that these cleaners all contain different chemicals, and that by using four or five of them each day we expose ourselves to high levels of toxins.

HAZARDOUS TO HEALTH

There are a number of cleaning-related chemicals and compounds that should be avoided in the home. Be aware that many of them never make it onto the labels of cleaning products.

VOCs: Volatile organic compounds are used as performance enhancers. Released as gases from certain liquids or solids, they can affect neurological function.

Phthalates: These compounds, which distribute dyes and fragrances in cleaners, may cause harmful hormonal effects.

Phospates: Used to disperse dirt and grease in laundry and dish detergents, these chemicals deplete oxygen in rivers and lakes when they enter the water supply.

To begin your wellness revamp, assess each room in the house, looking for questionable products. Check the kitchen for counter cleaners; glass cleaners; bottles or containers made of #3, #6, or #7 plastics; and flaking Teflon pans. Check the bathroom for harsh cleansers, liquid soap, air fresheners, and cosmetics with parabens. Scope out the laundry area for detergents and dryer sheets. In all cases, consider replacing risky products with safe, green alternatives. Also watch out for polyurethane foam (found in many mattresses), which emits VOCs, and fabrics treated with flame-retardants, which may cause nervous system disorders and cancer.

PANTRY PRIDE

There are multiple benefits to using the following time-tested natural cleaners: they are safe, effective, inexpensive, and probably already right in your home.

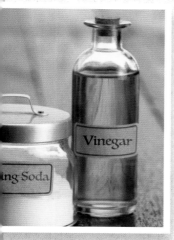

Baking soda and vinegar

Vinegar: The wellness and green communities have rediscovered this age-old body tonic and employ it as a disinfectant, a deodorizer, and a surface cleaner that makes stainless steel gleam.

Lemon: The naturally acidic juice of lemons provides a powerful cleaning and disinfecting agent that also provides a bright citrus scent.

Baking Soda: This stomach settler and deodorizer also makes a great kitchen and bath scrub. Use it on porcelain, tile, and metal surfaces to remove grease and grime.

Salts: These abrasive crystals can be used as scouring agents, and to clear gummy sink drains, polish tarnished metal, remove water rings on wood, and degrease pots and pans.

Pest Controls: There are plenty of herbs and botanicals, such as neem and geranium oil, pennyroyal, lavender, and peppermint, that will repel moths, fleas, ticks, roaches, mosquitoes, mice, and other crawling and flying nuisances in the home and garden.

SAFE ALTERNATIVES

Air fresheners that produce VOCs can be replaced by herbal options—potpourris, sachets, essential oil diffusers, but not by scented candles, which leave chemicals and soot behind. Dryer sheets also give off VOCs and can be replaced by felt dryer balls, which prevent static and fluff laundry as it dries.

VINEGAR SOLUTIONS

Vinegar was valued as a cleaner and light disinfectant for thousands of years. Happily, it has recently been rediscovered as a child- and pet-safe, chemical-free option for cleaning kitchen and bath surfaces.

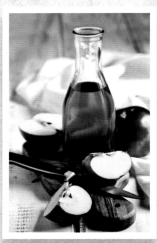

Apple cider vinegar

The concept of using fermented fruit to make vinegar goes back at least to 5000 BC, when the Babylonians made wine and vinegar from dates. From biblical times to the present, it has been drunk as an energizing tonic, prescribed as a remedy, and used as an astringent surface cleaner. Apple cider or white vinegar both make excellent cleaners; save the more expensive wine and balsamic vinegars to sprinkle on your salads.

VERSATILE DEGREASER

Vinegar's high level of acidity allows it to cut through grease and grime; it can even dissolve the soap scum and brine left by hard water. Combined with baking soda, it eliminates set red-wine stains. It is also safer than bleach for lightening stained fabrics. Although it can eradicate microorganisms, it does not destroy staphylococcus germs. Still, once you start replacing chemical cleaners and disinfectants with vinegar, you'll be surprised at how many uses you'll find for it.

Window Cleaner: To thoroughly clean your windows without harsh chemicals, make a mixture of equal parts distilled white vinegar and water. Spray your windows or apply with a sponge and wipe clean with a lint-free cloth or newspaper.

White vinegar and water make a good window cleaning solution

Tip: If you're using a squeegee to dry your windows, wet the blade before you use it so it won't skip.

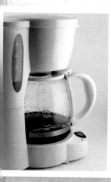

Cleanse Your Coffeemaker: Fill the reservoir of your coffeemaker with distilled white vinegar and run it through a brewing cycle to dissolve any old coffee buildup, mineral residue, and stains. Once the cycle is complete, empty the carafe and rinse any remaining vinegar by running another full brewing cycle with just water.

Cleanse your coffeemaker

Furniture Polish: To add a sheen to your wooden furniture, make your own polish using vinegar. Combine ¼ cup white vinegar with 1 cup olive oil to clean and condition wood furniture. You can add a few drops of lemon or orange oil for a deodorizing effect.

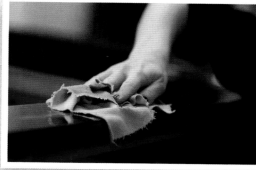

Make your own polish using vinegar

Clean Your Microwave: If you have food buildup in your microwave, combine ¼ cup white vinegar and 1 cup of water in a bowl. Place in the microwave and turn the microwave on until steam forms on the window. Then, after waiting for it to cool, remove the bowl and give the inside of your microwave a swipe—the residue should come straight off.

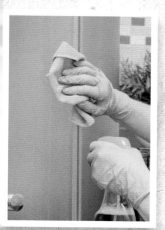

Maintain Shower Doors: To prevent soap-scum buildup on your shower doors or walls, wipe the surfaces with a sponge or rag soaked in white vinegar and let dry. Do not rinse or buff the vinegar away—this will allow grime to accumulate over time. Repeat this process regularly to easily maintain a clean shower.

Maintain shower doors

Floor Cleaner: For an effective floor cleaner that won't harm your pets or children, combine ½ cup white vinegar with a half gallon of warm water. This method is safe on tile, vinyl, and wooden floors alike.

Tip: Undiluted vinegar is acidic, so be sure to test this mixture on your floors in an unobtrusive place before use.

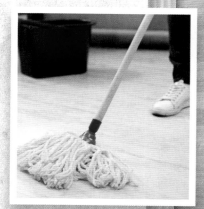

Floor cleaner

VINEGAR SOLUTIONS

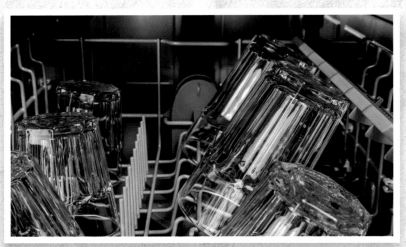

Add white vinegar to your dishwasher for sparklingly clean glassware

Sparkling Glasses: Add 1½ to 2 cups white vinegar to the bottom of your dishwasher for sparklingly clean glassware and dishes. Run your dishwasher on its regular cycle with your usual detergent.

Countertops: Make a mixture of equal parts white vinegar and water to easily clean your countertops. Simply spray or wipe the mixture onto the surface using a rag or sponge, and clean normally. Note: While vinegar is safe for most surfaces, it can cause pitting on countertops that are granite, marble, and soapstone. (To kill staphylococcus germs, use hydrogen peroxidem not vinegar).

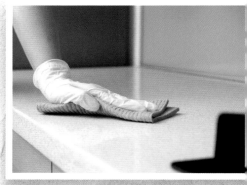

Clean countertops

Remove Tarnish: To remove tarnish from your copper, brass, and pewter cutlery or kitchenware, make a paste with 1 teaspoon salt, ½ cup white vinegar, and ½ teaspoon flour. Apply this mixture to the metal and let it sit for 15 minutes. Rinse with water, and polish with a soft, dry cloth.

Tip: Avoid using paper towels to polish your metalware, as they can scratch the surface.

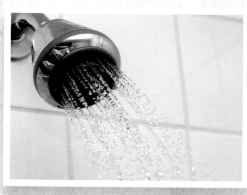

Keep your showerhead clean

Clogged Showerhead: Mineral buildup in showerheads can occur over time, especially if the water in your area is hard. This buildup affects the water pressure and the overall quality of your shower. To dissolve this buildup, fill a small plastic bag with vinegar and position the bag so the showerhead sits in the vinegar. Use a rubber band to hold the bag in place and let it sit overnight. Once you have removed the bag, run your shower to remove any buildup or remaining vinegar.

Fabric Softener: Add a cup of white vinegar to your laundry during the final wash of your laundry cycle to soften your clothes and remove static cling. It's a cheap way to get soft, clean clothes while helping to protect the environment from VOC-laden dryer sheets.

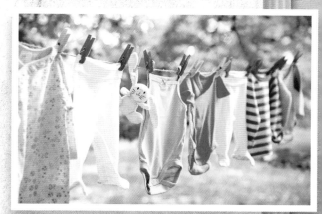

Add white vinegar to your wash to soften your clothes

Clean Your Tub: Remove dingy film from your tub by using baking soda and vinegar. Spray or wipe the surfaces with white vinegar and then sprinkle baking soda over the same area. Rinse away with clean water. For more stubborn grime, let the vinegar and baking soda sit for a few minutes, or add some elbow grease and buff the spot with a bristle brush or damp sponge.

Cutting Boards: To clean and sanitize your cutting boards, simply spray the surface with undiluted white vinegar, wipe, and rinse clean.
Tip: For wooden cutting boards that will last a long time, follow up with mineral oil or a food-safe wood oil to seal and protect the wood.

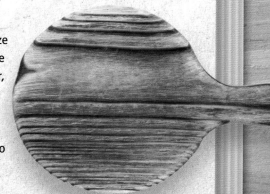

Clean and sanitize your cutting boards

LEMON SOLUTIONS

This sunny citrus fruit with the bright aroma and sour taste also provides powerful antibacterial properties—making it ideal for cleaning and disinfecting surfaces in both the kitchen and bathroom.

YOUR MAIN SQUEEZE

Lemon oil is often referred to as "liquid sunshine"; it also happens to be the most effective antimicrobial remedy of all essential oils. But the juice of the lemon is also a powerful bacteria eliminator, even diluted. Straight up, it cuts through dried-on cheese, bleaches tough stains, unclogs drains . . . you can even use it to sanitize the silver or stainless-steels posts of earrings.

DIY: Lemony All-purpose Cleaner

The acidity of lemons makes them a great option for all kinds of cleaning. Prepare a powerful all-purpose cleaner for daily use with just lemons, white vinegar, and water. In a glass jar or a clear plastic spray bottle, mix 2 cups of white vinegar, 2 cups of water, and the juice and rinds of ½ a lemon. Leave the mixture to sit for about 2 weeks in a cool spot out of direct sunlight, and then transfer the liquid to a spray bottle. For best results, wait for a few seconds after spraying before wiping it away, to give the cleaner time to work.

Clean and Deodorize Garbage Disposals: Garbage disposals are convenient and useful parts of our kitchens, but they also attract odors and bacteria. And cleaning them is not as easy as the other surfaces in your kitchen—it can even be dangerous. Fortunately, there is an easy, natural way to deodorize your garbage disposal and kill the bacteria that can live in it. Make deodorizing pods by mixing ¾ cup baking soda, ½ cup table salt, ½ teaspoon of dish soap, and the zest of 1 lemon. Add lemon juice until the mixture looks like slightly wet sand (about 3 tablespoons of juice). Pack tightly into an empty ice cube tray and allow to dry overnight. Remove pods and store in an airtight container. When ready to use, drop one pod into the garbage disposal and turn on. Use as needed to keep your garbage disposal clean and odor free.

Clean Glass: From mirrors to windows to sliding patio doors, glass is everywhere in our houses, and if you have small children or pets, these glass objects never seem to stay smudge free. Store-bought glass cleaners are full of harsh chemicals and dyes that can be dangerous to your family, especially

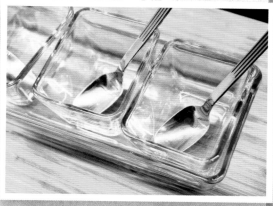

Clean glass

if you use them often. These chemicals can also be dangerous to other, nonglass surfaces in your house. There is a natural, effective alternative, however, one you can make using lemon juice. Simply add 3 tablespoons of lemon juice and ½ cup of rubbing alcohol to a spray bottle. Fill rest of the bottle with water and shake well to mix.

Clean Toilets: Toilet bowls are one of the germiest places in a home, and keeping them clean can be a real chore. Commercial toilet cleaners are also one of the most dangerous home cleaners—they cause burns if they get on your skin, plus the fumes can be harmful for you and your family. A less-dangerous solution can be made using lemon juice and borax. Sprinkle ¼ cup of borax into the toilet bowl and then squeeze in half a lemon. Let the mixture sit in the bowl for a few minutes. Scrub with a brush, then flush.

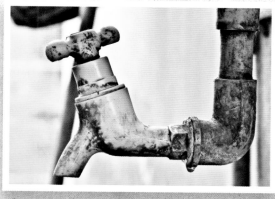

Scour rust

Scour Rust: As metal objects get older, they tend to rust. This is unsightly and unsafe, especially when the rust is on kitchen appliances. Rust is notoriously difficult to remove, and commercial rust cleaners are full of dangerous chemicals. Scraping the rust off can cause the rust to get into the air and be breathed in accidentally. Luckily, all you really need to remove oxidation is a lemon and some coarse salt. Rub a liberal amount of salt over the rusted area. Squeeze or spray lemon juice over the whole area, and allow to sit for about 3 hours. Then, scrub the area with lemon rinds to remove the rust.

LEMON SOLUTIONS

Remove Sweat Stains: White T-shirts are particularly prone to getting unsightly yellow sweat stains that can seem impossible to remove. Often, commercial stain removers will not work for these types of stains, and using bleach can ruin other clothes in the wash. Lemon juice, however, can work as a bleaching agent without ruining your laundry. All you need to do is fill a spray bottle with pure, undiluted lemon juice. Before washing a shirt with sweat stains, spray the stains thoroughly with the lemon juice. Then, wash the shirt as you would normally, and the stains should fade.

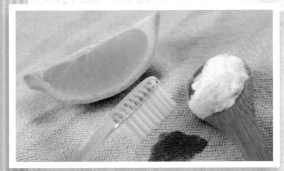

Mix baking soda and lemon to create an effective cleaner

Deodorize Carpets: Make your own carpet deodorizer by combining 2 cups of baking soda with 20 drops of lemon essential oil. Sprinkle the mixture over the whole carpet and allow to sit for about 15 minutes, longer for dirtier carpets. Then, simply vacuum up the powder and enjoy your fresh carpet. Store in a shaker jar for easy use.

Tip: For an even fresher scent, add about 5 drops of another essential oil, such as thyme or rosemary, to the mixture.

Whiten Clothes: Traditional methods of whitening clothes by using chlorine-based bleach can be dangerous and harmful to your health. Bleach fumes should not be breathed in, and if bleach gets on your skin, it can cause painful irritation. It also smells terrible. Many bleach products have fragrances added to try to mask the smell,

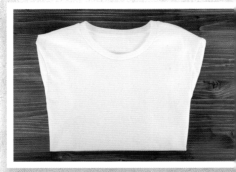

Whiten clothes

and these fragrances can stay in your clothes and cause irritation when you wear them. Lemon juice, on the other hand, is a natural alternative to chlorine bleach that smells great and is far less dangerous. Simply add ¼ cup of lemon juice to your white wash during the rinse cycle. Dry the clothes in the sun to activate the brightening effects of the lemon juice.

Clean Microwave: Place half a lemon, cut side up, in a bowl. Fill bowl with water and place in the microwave. Microwave on high for 5 minutes. Grime and stains should easily wipe off the inside surface of the microwave. If they do not, microwave the bowl for another 5 minutes. Tip: add 20 drops of your favorite essential oil to the water before microwaving to deodorize the microwave.

Wash Fruits and Vegetables:
Fruits and vegetables that we buy from the grocery store are usually sprayed with pesticides and waxes to keep them fresh and looking nice. However, consuming these pesticides can make you and your family sick. To remove them before eating, simply mix 1 tablespoon of lemon juice with 2 tablespoons of baking soda and 1 cup of

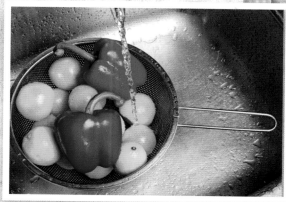

Wash fruits and vegetables

water. Whisk the mixture until the baking soda is completely dissolved. Pour the mixture into a spray bottle, then spray produce until it is completely soaked with the mixture. Let the mixture sit on the produce for about 5 minutes, then rinse thoroughly and dry.

Tip: Use this spray on organic produce and produce that you grow yourself as well. While the organic produce may not be sprayed with pesticides, it could have bacteria on it that will be killed using this lemon-baking soda spray.

Clean Humidifiers: Even with regular cleaning, humidifiers can need a little extra treatment to prevent the growth of bacteria, mold, and mildew. A natural way to do this is by adding 1 tablespoon of fresh lemon juice to the water in the humidifier every time you fill it. The lemon juice will kill bacteria that can grow in the water and will release a pleasant scent into the air as well.

Clean Mildewed Clothes: Mildew can grow anywhere there is a damp place without ventilation, such as a child's sports locker. It can be smelly and annoying, and sometimes mildew can be a hazard to your health. It might seem impossible to remove from fabric, and you might be tempted to just throw the item away. There is a natural solution for this problem, however. Due to its antifungal properties, lemon juice works very well at removing mildew. Simply add salt to ⅓ cup of fresh lemon juice to form a paste, then rub the paste into the fabric. If necessary, scrub the paste in using an old toothbrush. Then, wash the fabric as normal.

BAKING SODA SOLUTIONS

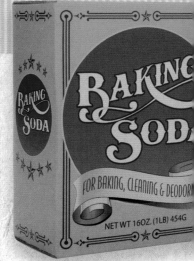

This household staple has a variety of handy uses, a lot more than its usual job of sitting in the refrigerator keeping bad odors away. It can even clear backed-up drains, with a little help from vinegar.

THE GREAT CLEANER IN A LITTLE BOX

Baking soda, or sodium bicarbonate, has many traditional health applications—antacid, mouthwash, deodorant—but it is also an effective cleaner and scrub. A similar substance, sodium carbonate, was used around 3500 BC as a soap-like cleaning agent—and to help make mummies! Baking soda was created in 1843 by British chemist Alfred Bird, whose wife had an allergy to yeast. It is made of two minerals, nahcolite and trona, which are refined into soda ash (calcium carbonate), then into sodium bicarbonate. Most of the raw materials come from the United States.

DIY: Easy Dishwasher Detergent

By making your own detergent with baking soda, you will eliminate unwanted grease and grime from your dishes and lower the amount of harmful chemicals used in your home. Add 3 drops of regular dish soap to your dishwasher's detergent cup, then fill the cup two thirds of the way up with baking soda. Fill the remaining space in the cup with sea salt, and run your dishwasher as normal. .

Remove Stains from Plastic Containers: Wipe your food storage containers with a clean sponge sprinkled with baking soda. For tougher stains, soak the containers in a solution of 4 teaspoons of baking soda to a quart of warm water.

Deodorize Your Kitchen: Baking soda is a powerful deodorizer that will absorb strong food odors. Just as it will deodorize your refrigerator, baking soda can do wonders for your garbage can. Pour a layer of baking soda into the bottom of your trash can to fight any lingering odors.

Clean Kitchen Surfaces: Sprinkle baking soda onto a clean, damp sponge or cloth and clean as usual. Rinse thoroughly and wipe dry. This method is safe on all kitchen surfaces.

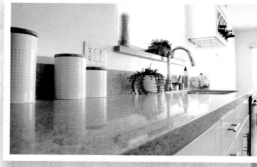

Clean kitchen surfaces

Tip: For a deeper clean, make a paste with baking soda, coarse salt, and liquid dish soap to scour tough grime. Give your surfaces a wipe with a cloth dampened with distilled white vinegar and water to remove any streaks left by the baking soda.

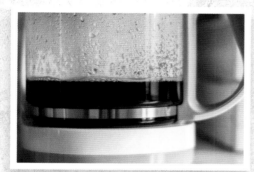

Clean your coffeepot

Clean Your Coffeepot: Mix ¼ cup baking soda with 1 quart warm water. Rub the mixture in and on your pots to remove stains or to eliminate bad tastes from your coffee- or teapot. In the case of tough stains, let the mixture sit for a few hours and then rinse.

Clean Silverware: Create a paste of three parts baking soda to one part water. Apply this with a lint-free cloth; let sit for 15 to 20 minutes, then rinse.

Tip: Avoid using paper towels to apply the mixture, as they can scratch your silverware.

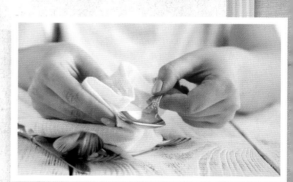

Clean silverware

Degrease Ovens: To effectively clean your oven, simply add a teaspoon of baking soda to a damp rag or sponge to wipe away any food or grease remnants without using harmful chemicals. For stubborn messes on your pots and pans, add a sprinkle of baking soda to whatever pan you're cleaning to dissolve stuck-on grease and add more abrasive scouring power.

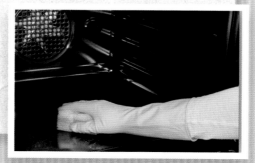

BAKING SODA SOLUTIONS

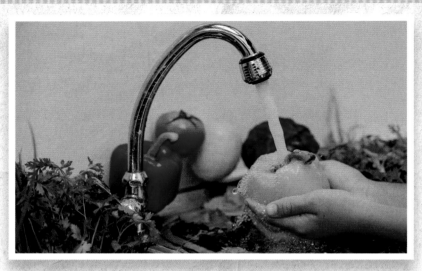

Scrub Your Veggies: Baking soda is a food-safe way to remove any dirt or pesticide residue off fresh fruit and vegetables. Just sprinkle some baking soda onto a damp cloth, wipe your produce, and rinse.

Remove mildew: Scrub your tub, tile, sink, and shower curtain with a damp sponge and baking soda for a healthy way to keep your bathroom clean.

Unclog a Drain: Pour a ½ cup of baking soda down your drain and follow with a ½ cup of white vinegar to re-create your science class "volcano" project in your kitchen or bathroom. Cover with a wet cloth to contain the reaction. Wait 5 minutes and then flush with hot water to clear the drain. This method will work on any mild clog.

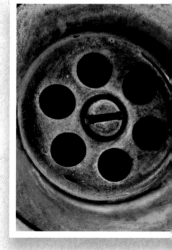

Shower Curtain Cleaner: Wipe shower curtains and plastic liners with a damp cloth or sponge sprinkled with baking soda and rinse to remove grime and soap scum.

Cat Litter Deodorizer: Cover the bottom of your cat's litter box before filling it with litter as usual to naturally deodorize it. After adding the litter and after each time you clean out the litter, sprinkle extra baking soda on top for a deodorizing boost.

Septic Care: If your home has a septic tank, you'll know that maintaining it is very important and any issues with the tank can be problematic and costly to repair. Flushing 1 cup of baking soda per week will keep your septic system functioning well and maintain a good pH balance in your septic tank.

Clean Smooth Surfaces: Sprinkle baking soda onto a clean damp sponge or cloth and clean kitchen sinks, surrounds, counters, and the refrigerator exterior. Rinse thoroughly, and wipe dry.

DIY: All-purpose Floor Cleaner
This natural floor cleaner is safe for wood, vinyl, and tile floors alike and removes any lingering smells. Combine ¼ cup white vinegar, ¼ cup baking soda, 1 teaspoon liquid dish soap, 2 gallons warm water.

Tip: For a deeper clean, make a paste with baking soda. Using a sponge or cloth, rub the mixture onto the surface you want to clean. Let it sit for 15–20 minutes and then wipe with a cloth to scour tough grime.

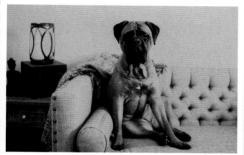

Deodorize Musty Upholstery: Children and pets can make it hard to maintain your furniture, particularly larger items such as sofas. For upholstered furniture pieces that don't have removable covers, try using baking soda as a way to keep them fresh. Sprinkle any fabric surfaces in your home with baking soda. Let it sit for 15 minutes, then vacuum.
Tip: You can use this method on your mattress as well as your pets' beds.

Remove Crayon from Walls: Don't want to repaint every time your kid moves his crayon from paper to the walls? Scrub lightly with a damp sponge sprinkled with baking soda to remove crayon or pencil marks from most surfaces. As baking soda is lightly abrasive, test this method on an unobtrusive area of the wall to ensure that it won't damage the finish of the paint.

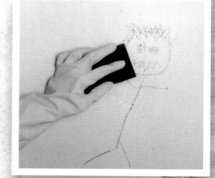

Buff Out Water Rings: Make a paste of one part baking soda to one part water. Apply this to any water rings left on your wooden surfaces and gently buff the stain away.

BAKING SODA SOLUTIONS

Carpet Cleaner: Many carpet cleaners contain chemicals that are harmful to children and pets—baking soda is a natural way to keep your home clean while keeping your family healthy. Sprinkle your carpet

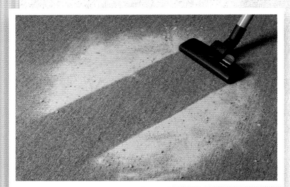

thoroughly with baking soda; let it sit for 15–20 minutes, then vacuum. For a deeper clean, spray the stained area with a 1:1 mixture of white vinegar and water. Wait up to an hour, or until the surface dries, then scrub the baking soda loose and vacuum.

Clean your carpets

Brighten Your Laundry: Add a cup of baking soda to your laundry load to brighten whites and colors alike. When combined with liquid detergent, baking soda will help balance the pH levels to give clothes a more thorough clean. Use one cup of baking soda alone in your laundry for a gentle way to clean and soften baby clothes.

Deodorize Sneakers: Sprinkle some baking soda inside your shoes (and your gym bag) to minimize odor. Leave until your next wear, just be sure to shake out the excess before you put them on.

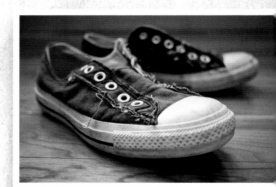

Deodorize sneakers

Remove Stains: Make a thick paste of baking soda and water (4 tablespoons baking soda with ¼ cup water). Rub the paste into the stain, let it sit for an hour, and launder as usual to remove perspiration stains. This mixture is also effective for removing rust stains and fresh grease stains. For general stain removal, let the baking soda mixture sit for 3 hours before washing. For fresh coffee and wine stains, soak the area in white vinegar and dab with a clean towel, then sprinkle baking soda over the stain and rub with a clean, soft toothbrush before laundering in cold water. For oil stains, add a drizzle of dish soap over the baking soda before brushing the stain and laundering in cold water.

Improve Your Linen Closet: Place an open box or bowl of baking soda in your linen closet to fight musty smells in your sheets and towels. **Tip:** This also works for your bedroom closets!

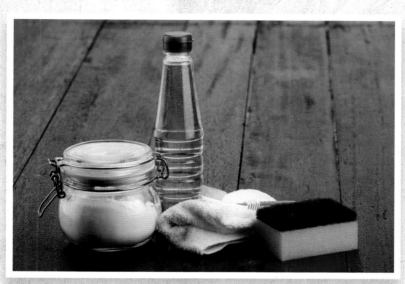

Bakings soda

Freshen Your Hamper: Sprinkle baking soda into the bottom of your clothes hamper to keep odors away; over time, a cloth hamper can absorb the odors of what it contains.

Clean Your Iron: To ensure that you do not leave lime stains or marks on your light-colored clothes, give your iron a clean using white vinegar and baking soda. Soak a piece of paper towel or clean cloth with vinegar, then sprinkle baking soda over the cloth. Place the iron on the cloth and move in circular motions (make sure the iron is turned off). Once it's clean, turn the iron on and set it to steam setting to remove any baking soda from the iron's holes. Repeat this process until your iron is clean.

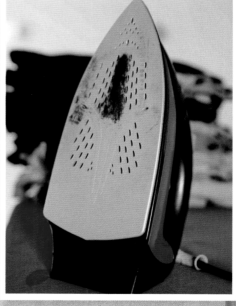

Clean your iron

SALT SOLUTIONS

For millennia salt was a rare and valuable commodity—the word "salary" comes from the Roman habit of paying soldiers in salt. Today it is plentiful, and has become more than just a condiment or means of curing meats.

Salt, or sodium chloride, comes from two sources: sea water or the mineral halite, also called rock salt. In ancient Rome, roads were built specifically to bring the mineral to the capital. Since medieval times salt has been used as a cleaner, and with its nontoxic yet abrasive character, it is still popular for scouring surfaces and removing stains around the house. It is also a catalyst to boost the cleaning and deodorizing power of other cleaners like vinegar.

Salt

CLEAN STAINED CLOTHES

Try these tricks to get different types of stubborn stains out of fabrics.

Blood stains: Salt and water make an efficient and cost-effective way to remove blood stains from fabrics. You can either rub dry salt into the stain first and then soak the garment in cold water, or you can simply soak the whole thing in a saltwater bath. Follow up with a soap-and-water wash, and finally rinse with warm—not hot—water.

Tip: Don't use hot water at first—it may set the stain deeper rather than washing it out. Also, using seltzer instead of tap water can be even more effective.

Wine Stains: When removing red wine stains from your clothes, it's best to start as soon as possible after the spill so that the stain doesn't set. Blot the stain dry as much as you can without rubbing the wine further into the fabric. Then, cover the stain with salt, allowing it to break up the stain and absorb as much of it as possible. Let it sit for a few minutes, then wash the garment with soap and warm water.

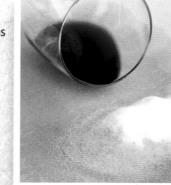

Clean wine stains

Sweat Stains: To wash sweat stains or yellowing out of clothes, soak the fabric for several minutes in a solution of 4 tablespoons of salt for every quart of hot water. Let soak for several minutes and then wash as you otherwise would, and all discoloration should vanish.

Pots and Pans: To clean greasy or food-crusted pans, use a mixture of salt and vinegar to scour away unwanted debris. Pour salt and white vinegar into the pan and swish around until the food and grease come loose. Rinse the pan, then clean as normal.

Tip: Use a rough sponge to help scrub away any hard-to-clean food residue.

Clean Up Raw Egg: If you spill a raw egg on the floor or kitchen counter while cooking, you can use salt to make the cleanup a little easier. Pouring salt on the egg before you wipe it up should make the egg coagulate, making the job easier and less messy.

Clean a Stained Bathtub: Salt can be used as an inexpensive scrub to remove stains from the bathtub. Mix equal parts salt and turpentine to form a paste, then scrub stains from tub. The stains will lift quickly and easily. Using a washcloth or a firm sponge in combination with this cleaning solution should be enough to scour even deep stains without damaging your bathtub.

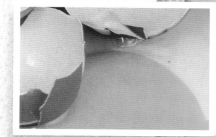

Clean egg spills

Unclog a Drain: If your kitchen sink is clogged with food residue, pour ¼ cup baking soda and ¼ cup salt into a clogged drain, followed by ½ cup of white vinegar. Let sit for about 20 minutes, then follow with a pot of boiling water. If the drain isn't completely cleared after this, repeating the process should produce the desired results.

Clean a Refrigerator: To clean your refrigerator's shelves and drawers after emptying it out—or to clean up after a spill—you can use a mixture of salt and seltzer water. The coarse texture of the salt will help scrub off any food residue or stubborn stains, as well as deodorize your fridge for future use.

Clean Oven Spills: Salt is great for soaking up grease from stains and loosening accumulated grime on kitchen surfaces. This, combined with its abrasive nature, makes it a great choice when cleaning greasy stove tops or ovens. Start by applying a damp cloth to the area in question, then pour a liberal amount of salt wherever you can see stains. Leave it there for several minutes to clump over the mess and make it easier to clean, and then wipe the area down with another damp cloth or sponge.

NATURAL PEST CONTROL

Even the cleanest homes and neatest yards are beset by flying, creeping, and crawling pests every so often. Don't run for the chemical sprays, however—let natural deterrents and essential oils get the job done.

DON'T BUG ME

There are plenty of safe methods to convince insects, mice, and other unwelcome critters to stay clear of you, your pets, your home, and your backyard.

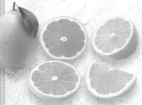

The smell of lemons can help repel ants

Lemon for Ants: The smell of lemons can help repel ants. The lemon scent will cover the scent tracks they use to communicate where to go. There are three methods for preventing ants from entering your home and pantries: Soak a washcloth in lemon juice and wipe down all areas where you think ants are entering the house. Leave lemon rinds around outside doorways to repel them. Soak cotton balls with lemon essential oil and place in cabinets where food is kept.

Keep Ants Out with Salt: One way to deal with an ant problem—without setting down traps or poison that could harm pets or small children—is to line doorways and windowsills with salt. Sprinkle a line of salt anywhere you suspect ants or other insects may be entering your house, and you should see a noticeable decrease in the number of ants in your home.

Mice Deterrent: In order to counter any unwelcome rodent visitors, sprinkle borax on the floor along the walls and on any areas where you believe the mice may be entering your home. Mice tend to run along the floor at the base of walls but dislike getting borax on their feet and therefore are less likely to return to that area of the house. Peppermint sachets are also quite effective: mice hate the smell and will avoid it at all costs.

Flea Killer: If you suspect that you have fleas breeding in your home, try using borax to eliminate the problem. Identify any and all areas where fleas might be hatching, and sprinkle a light layer of borax over the area. Let the borax sit on there for a day and then vacuum it away. Good places to check are dog beds, carpets, and any other areas where pets gather in your home.

Pest-free Pets: You can keep Fido flea and tick free by using natural controls. Slice a lemon, place it in a bowl, then pour boiling water over it and let it soak overnight. Sponge the liquid over your dog's coat to give fleas the brush. (Do not use on cats.) Make a pennyroyal or cedar antiflea sachet to attach to your dog's collar. Or make one with geranium oil to repel ticks.

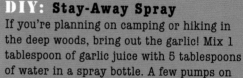

DIY: Stay-Away Spray

If you're planning on camping or hiking in the deep woods, bring out the garlic! Mix 1 tablespoon of garlic juice with 5 tablespoons of water in a spray bottle. A few pumps on exposed skin will keep hungry flying insects away for hours.

Personal Repellents: You can keep mosquitoes away from family and friends outdoors with applications of the essential oils of lemongrass, sage, or rosemary. You can also purchase nontoxic pheromone mosquito traps to hang in the yard.

Tip: Diatomaceous earth sprinkled in outdoor play areas will help discourage ticks from preying on children and pets.

Keep Out Pests: If you are dealing with an infestation of roaches or ants, simply make a mixture of equal parts sugar and borax and sprinkle the mixture anywhere you think the insects may be entering your home.

Kill Cockroaches: Many of the commercial options for dealing with a cockroach infestation are loaded with harmful chemicals. Fortunately, a more natural option is available: you can kill cockroaches with white vinegar. Put white vinegar in a spray bottle and spray roaches whenever you see them. Additionally, you should wipe down your floors and countertops with white vinegar to clean the surfaces and remove any lingering smells of foods or crumbs that attract roaches and other pests.

YOUR HEALTHY HOME CHECKLIST

Here is a handy list to follow to make sure you are doing your best to keep your family safe and your home green. Take a few steps in the right direction, and eliminating toxins will soon become second nature.

A quick sweep through your house will allow you to assess potential health risks that may be lurking in the guise of cleaners, air fresheners, and bug sprays. If you're concerned about the environment and conservation, you should also pay attention to "green" issues, such as maintaining heating and cooling units at the proper temperatures. And by changing batteries and filters in a timely manner, you are ensuring that alarms for safety hazards are functional and that airborne pathogens will continue to be banished from your home.

THE BIG PICTURE
Making the following changes will absolutely improve the quality of your life and home.

Eliminate VOCs: As much as is possible, rid your home of volatile organic compounds, including plug-in air fresheners, dryer sheets, acetone nail polish remover, bug sprays, and, perhaps the worst of the lot, household cleaners, which expose people to a variety of toxins on a daily basis. Clean is not necessarily green. (And, as you have seen in this chapter, there are far healthier cleaning and disinfecting alternatives.)

DON'T DUMP HAZARDOUS WASTE:
Never flush any chemicals down the drain. Remove old paint cans, used motor oil, weed and bug killers, and other harsh chemicals from the garage and basement at least once a year. Don't throw out old batteries or electronics. Your community should have designated drop-off sites or monthly waste pickup to safely dispose of these hazards.

Banish Formaldehyde: If you are buying new wooden furniture, especially from a big-box store, make sure it is formaldehyde free; this is particularly important for baby furniture. Vintage wooden furniture is a good alternative—any formaldehyde used in its manufacture is long gone.

Stop Mold: Mold will grow where there is moisture and food, such as on damp paper. Make sure to check around plumbing fixtures for leaks and around windows for condensation that can cause mold. Keep humidity levels down in the winter.

Add Indoor Plants: Houseplants have the ability to absorb carbon dioxide and formaldehyde and to produce oxygen. They are helpful for filtering the air in today's tightly sealed homes and office buildings.

Take Off Your Shoes: This is important if you have young children who crawl on the floor. Studies show that toxins such as pesticides are carried in on footwear and deposited on rugs and carpets, where toddlers are exposed to them to a surprising degree.

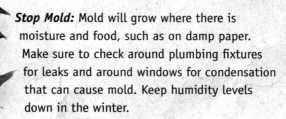

Houseplant

TIMELY INSPECTIONS

Batteries: Make sure you change the batteries in smoke detectors and carbon-monoxide detectors at the spring and fall equinox in March and September. Older car batteries should be checked in fall to make sure they are retaining the proper charge.

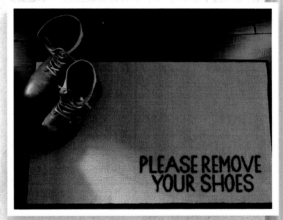

PLEASE REMOVE YOUR SHOES

Filters: Be sure to check your furnace and air-conditioner filters at the start of each usage season; check kitchen and bathroom exhaust fan filters and air-purifier filters every few months.

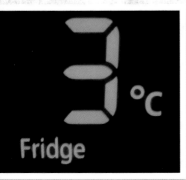

Temperatures: Maintain your refrigerator temperature around 37 degrees, and your freezer at -3 degrees. An electronic thermostat will instruct your furnace to heat your home at lower temps at night. In winter, set it for 68 during the day and 55 at night. In summer, keep your air conditioner at 78. Most water heaters work best between 120 and 140 degrees.

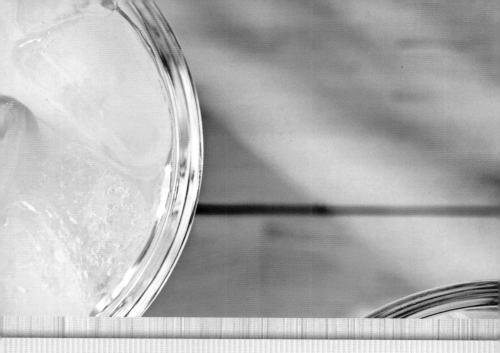

CHAPTER 8

TEAS, TONICS, AND SMOOTHIES

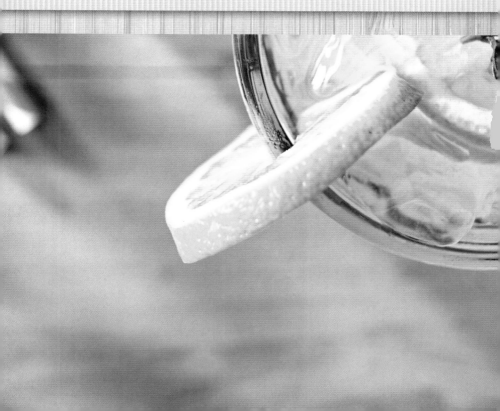

TEAS, TONICS, AND SMOOTHIES

It's just as easy to prepare a healthy beverage as it is to brew a cup of caffeinated coffee or to mix up a sugar-laden summer cooler. If you keep a few natural ingredients and some fresh produce on hand, you'll find that making healthy beverages is a breeze, whether you're brewing hot or iced teas, preparing healing tonics, or blending delicious, antioxidant fruit and vegetable smoothies.

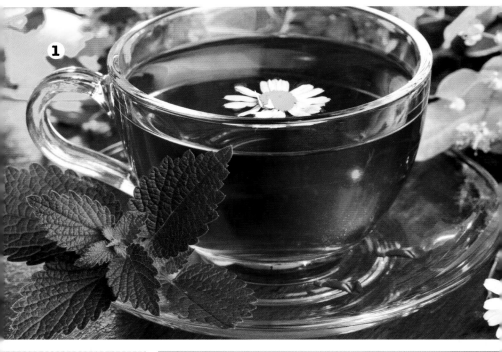

1 Sleep Tight Tea
2 Potent Ginger Turmeric Tea
3 Lemon Basil Iced Tea
4 Lavender-Lemon tonic
5 Anti-Bloat Spice Tonic
6 Berry Belly-Fat–Blaster Smoothie

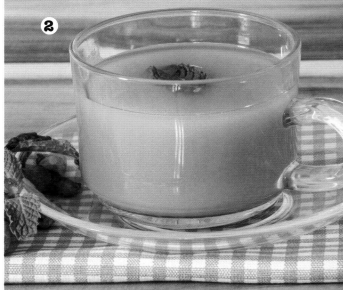

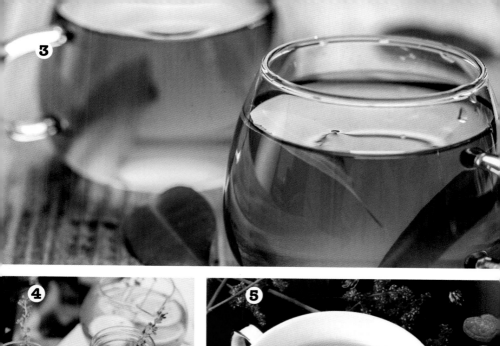

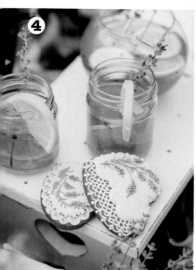

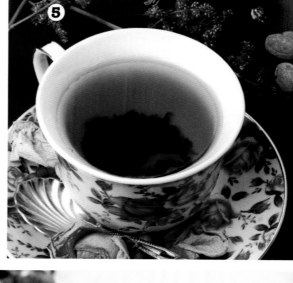

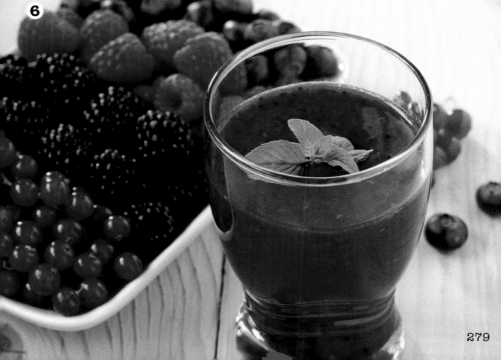

RESTORATIVE HOT TEAS

Potent Ginger-Turmeric Tea

Ingredients

• 2 cups water • ½ teaspoon ground turmeric • ½ teaspoon chopped fresh ginger • ½ teaspoon ground cinnamon • 1 tablespoon honey • 1 wedge of lemon

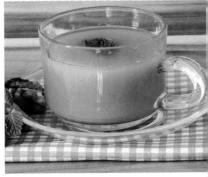

Turmeric Tea

Directions

• *In a saucepan, bring water to a boil.*
• *Add spices and reduce to medium heat; simmer for 10 minutes.*
• *Strain and serve with honey and lemon wedge. Or substitute real maple syrup for the honey.*

Benefits: This tea makes an excellent tonic, especially for those recovering from an illness. Turmeric is known for its restorative and preventative properties; it contains antioxidants and anti-inflammatories and offers antiseptic and analgesic benefits. Ginger calms digestion, eases the pain of arthritis, and treats respiratory conditions; it is used in more than 50 percent of traditional herbal remedies.

Traditional Masala Chai

Ingredients

• 1 cup water • 1½ teaspoons sugar • 1 whole green cardamom pod • 1 whole clove • 2 black peppercorns • 3 teaspoons black tea leaves • ½ cup warm milk

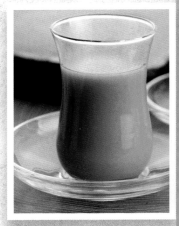

Traditional Masala Chai

Directions

• *Combine water and sugar in a small pan and bring to a boil.*
• *Add the spices and tea leaves. Remove from heat.*
• *Let the tea steep for 3 minutes, then strain into a cup.*
• *Fill the rest of the cup with milk.*

Benefits: This is a quick version of the traditional spicy chai prepared in India. It is good for soothing a nervous stomach. Cardamom, a member of the ginger family, is known for easing tooth pain, indigestion, and urinary problems, and helping to combat depression. Black tea is loaded with antioxidants and can help boost heart health, decrease risk of diabetes, and lower stress levels.

Spiced Vanilla Tea

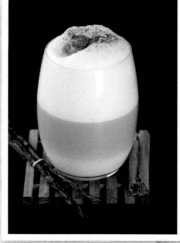

Ingredients
- 1 cup boiling water • 1 orange pekoe tea bag • 2 tablespoons milk • ½ teaspoon vanilla extract • ½ teaspoon ground cinnamon • 1 cinnamon stick

Directions
- *Pour boiling water into a mug and steep the tea bag for 3 minutes; discard tea bag.*
- *Add milk, vanilla, and cinnamon to the tea and stir.*
- *Garnish with a cinnamon stick.*

Spiced Vanilla Tea

Benefits: This is another take on chai tea, but with the addition of sweet vanilla. It makes a good wake-up beverage, but is a tasty treat any time of day. Cinnamon is known for aiding digestion and circulation, easing coughs and colds, calming muscle spasms, lowering blood sugar, and improving cognition. An extract found in the spice may inhibit the onset of Alzheimer's disease. Orange pekoe tea is a grade of black tea, which is known for providing antioxidant protection.

Green Tea with Citrus

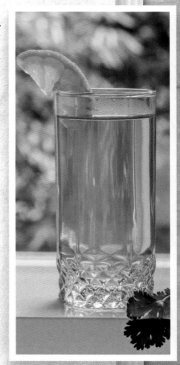

Ingredients
- Zest of 1 lemon wedge cut into slivers • 2 teaspoons boiling water • 2 teaspoons green tea powder • ¾ cup hot water • ½ cup fresh grapefruit or orange juice • 3 tablespoons fresh lemon juice • 1 teaspoon honey

Directions
- *Place lemon zest in mug and cover with 2 teaspoons boiling water.*
- *Steep for 3 minutes, then add green tea powder and hot water.*
- *Add fruit juice and honey; stir slightly.*

Benefits: The addition of fresh fruit juice adds vitamin C to this delightful, healthy tea. Teas in general are good for the heart, the circulatory system, and the immune system, and are full of antioxidants; green tea, specifically, has been linked to lowered risks for cancer.

Green Tea

RESTORATIVE HOT TEAS

Railroad Chai

Ingredients

- 2 cups water
- 1 tablespoon fennel seed
- 4 whole cloves, or more to taste
- 1½ teaspoons green cardamom seeds
- 2 cups whole milk
- 4 or 5 black tea bags
- 1 teaspoon sugar, or honey to taste

Directions

- *Boil water in a saucepan, then add spices. Boil for 3 minutes longer.*
- *Add milk and bring to a low boil, add tea bags, and lower heat.*
- *Simmer until tea is strong but not bitter.*
- *Strain into 4 mugs and sweeten to taste.*

Benefits: This is the familiar, beloved tea that is passed out on India's many railway lines. It has a distinctive flavor due to the use of fennel seeds. Its impressive health properties derive from three sources of antioxidants: fennel, tea, and cloves. Antioxidants boost the immune system and combat free radicals. Other benefits offered by this tea include antiviral, antibacterial, and anti-inflammatory qualities.

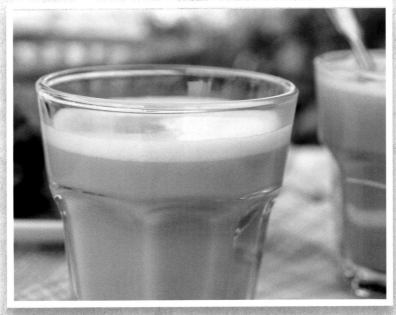

Railroad Chai

Spicy Citrus Cold Buster

Ingredients

• 6 cups hot water • 4-inch piece of fresh ginger, chopped coarsely • 1 whole star anise • 1 cinnamon stick • 6 green cardamom pods, bruised • 4 lemons • 3 tablespoons honey

Directions

• Bring the water to a boil in a saucepan, then add spices.
• Zest the lemon skin over the saucepan. Slice lemons in half and squeeze juice into the water.
• Reduce the heat to medium-low and simmer the mixture until it achieves a strong flavor, 5 to 15 minutes.
• Stir honey into tea and strain tea through a fine-mesh strainer as you pour into mugs. Makes 5 servings.
• Save spices left in strainer to reuse in your next batch of tea.

Benefits: This tea is perfect for treating winter ailments such as scratchy throats, stubborn coughs, and lingering colds. Its herbal components include respiratory-champ ginger, stomach-protecting and cholesterol-controlling cardamom, antioxidant and anti-inflammatory cinnamon, cough-relieving star anise, antiseptic honey, and astringent lemon juice.

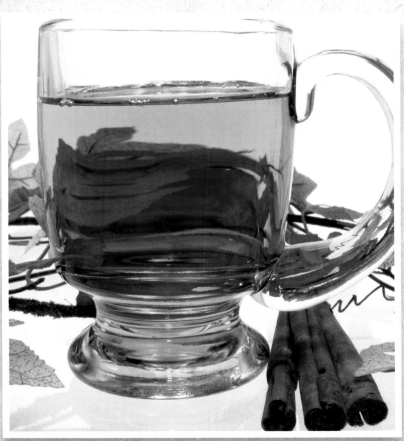

Spicy Citrus Cold Buster

RELAXING TEAS

Middle Eastern Tea

Ingredients
- 1½ cups water
- 1 sprig fresh or dried mint
- ½ sprig sage
- 2 Ceylon tea bags

Middle Eastern Tea

Directions
- *Add boiling water to mint and sage in teapot.*
- *Add tea bags and steep for 3 minutes.*
- *Sweeten with honey if necessary.*

Benefits: This tea will calm and relax you from breakfast time all the way through to the end of the day. Mint offers reliable, soothing support and calming agents for the stomach. Antioxidant sage strengthens the immune system and eliminates bloating and gas. Ceylon tea protects against chronic illnesses, boosts heart health, raises energy levels, and can aid in weight loss.

After-Dinner Licorice Tea

Ingredients
- ½ cup licorice root
- ¼ cup cinnamon chips
- ¼ cup dried orange peel
- ¼ cup dried ashwagandha
- ¼ cup astragalus root
- ¼ cup Siberian ginseng
- ¼ cup chamomile flowers
- 1 tablespoon dried cloves

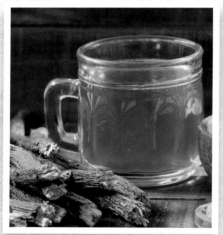

Directions
- *Mix herbs together and store in an airtight container.*
- *To make one cup, add 1 tablespoon of the mixture to one cup of boiling water and let steep for 15 to 30 minutes.*
- *Strain, reheat if necessary, and drink.*

After-Dinner Licorice Tea

Benefits: This flavorful digestive tea helps the stomach do its job, especially after a large meal. Licorice is known for relieving heartburn and easing anxiety. Cinnamon chips are small pieces of the bark; they add a warm flavor and support digestion. Ashwagandha and astragalus are both adaptogenic herbs that ease symptoms of stress. Siberian ginseng supports circulation and the immune system, anti-inflammatory chamomile relaxes muscles, and pungent cloves soothe the inner lining of the digestive tract.

Calming Lemon Tisane

Ingredients

- 3 parts lemongrass
- 1 part lemon balm
- 1 part lemon peel
- 1 part chamomile
- ⅛ part cut stevia leaf

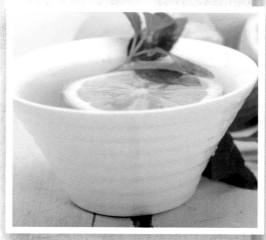

Calming Lemon Tisane

Directions

• *Add all the herbs to a glass jar and shake until they are completely mixed.*
• *Use one teaspoon of tisane for a single serving (about 8 oz). Add your desired amount to a tea strainer or teapot.*
• *Cover with boiling water a let steep for at least 5 minutes or up to 10.*
• *Sweeten with raw honey if desired.*

Child's Bedtime Tea

Ingredients

- 2 tablespoons raspberry leaves
- 2 tablespoons catnip
- 2 tablespoons spearmint leaves
- 1 tablespoon skullcap
- 2 tablespoons calendula flowers
- 1 pinch stevia

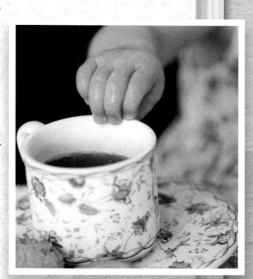

Child's Bedtime Tea

Directions

• *Mix herbal ingredients together in a lidded mason jar.*
• *Use 1 to 2 teaspoons per cup of boiling water.*
• *Let tea steep for 5 minutes, then strain, add stevia, and serve.*

Benefits: The gentle herbs that are combined in this tea make it ideal for serving to a restless child at bedtime or to an adult who is feeling under the weather. Raspberry is full of antioxidants that help battle cancer, heart disease, and aging. Catnip is a well-known calmative with analgesic properties. Spearmint improves digestion and circulation and boosts respiratory health. Skullcap is a traditional herbal remedy for anxiety and sleeplessness. Calendula is used to treat a sore throat or mouth and reduce swelling.

RELAXING TEAS

Antistress Herbal Tea

Ingredients
- 2½ cups boiling water
- 3 teaspoons chamomile flowers
- 2 teaspoons lemon balm
- 1 teaspoon skullcap
- 1 teaspoon lavender
- 1 big pinch peppermint
- 1 big pinch sage

Directions
• Place all ingredients in a teapot and pour boiling water over the contents.
• Allow the tea to steep for 3 to 5 minutes.
• Pour into cups through a strainer. Sweeten with honey if necessary. Serves 2

Benefits: This riot of herbal ingredients offer a very effective remedy for stress—chamomile and lavender are the relaxation champs of the herb world; lemon balm relieves stress, anxiety, and insomnia; peppermint eases digestion; and sage can reverse loss of appetite, reduce perspiration, and ease the symptoms of depression.

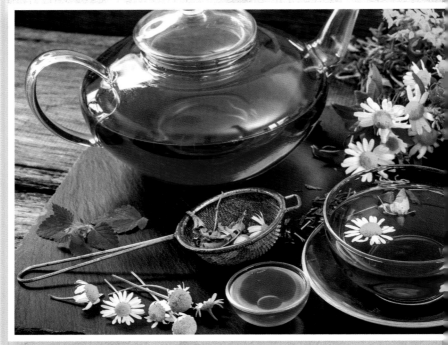

Anti-Stress Herbal Tea

Unbreak My Heart Tea

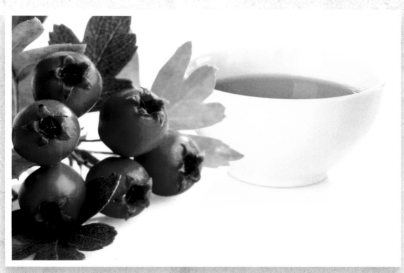

Unbreak My Heart Tea

Ingredients
- 1 teaspoon hawthorn leaf and flower
- 1 teaspoon motherwort
- ½ teaspoon passionflower

Directions
- *Blend the ingredients in a pot and add a cup of boiling water.*
- *Steep for 10 minutes, strain, and drink.*
- *Add honey to taste.*

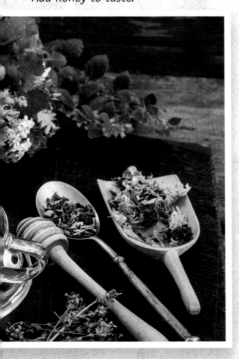

Benefits: This may be the elusive cure for a broken heart or grief over a loss (at least that's what some herbalists say). It's also a good calming tea. Hawthorn is known to regulate heartbeat and treat both high and low blood pressure. Motherwort relieves anxiety, treats insomnia, and helps control asthma. Passionflower is also used as a remedy for tension, anxiety, and sleeplessness.

THERAPEUTIC TEAS

Ultra Female-Hormone Balance

Ingredients
• 1 tablespoon alfalfa • 1 tablespoon red clover • 1 tablespoon raspberry leaf • 1 tablespoon yarrow • 1 tablespoon nettle • ½ tablespoon fennel seed • 1 tablespoon lemon balm • 1 tablespoon dried orange peel • 1 tablespoon hibiscus • 1 tablespoon peppermint or spearmint • 1 tablespoon chasteberry

Directions
• Blend the herbs and store in an airtight container.
• Use 1 teaspoon of dried herbs per cup of hot water.
• Cover and let steep for at least 20 minutes or up to 8 hours for a more potent infusion.
• Sweeten as desired with raw honey or stevia.
• Drink up to a quart, warm or at room temperature, throughout the day.

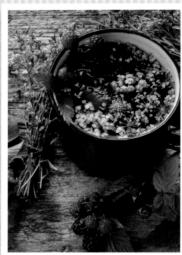

Ultra Female-Hormone Balance

Benefits: This blend works to balance hormones, reduce anxiety, and boost energy levels; it also doubles as a fertility tea. The alfalfa and red clover promote production of estrogen; raspberry leaf and yarrow are uterine tonics; nettle's bioavailable nutrients include calcium and magnesium; aromatic fennel seed is good for digestion; lemon balm lifts the spirits; orange peel is a catalyst herb that aids digestion; flavorful aromatic hibiscus furnishes vitamin C; peppermint and spearmint are uplifting and support digestion; and chasteberry helps balance hormones. Not to be taken during pregnancy.

Female-Ease Herbal Infusion

Ingredients
• 1 tablespoon white clover flowers • 1 tablespoon yarrow flowers
• 2 tablespoons raspberry leaves • 1 tablespoon lady's mantle leaves and flowers

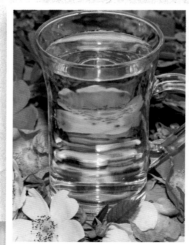

Directions
• *Combine the dried herbs in a quart-sized teapot.*
• *Fill with boiling water.*
• *Steep for 30 to 60 minutes, strain, and pour into mugs. Will keep in refrigerator for 2 days. Serves 2.*

Benefits: This tea helps to relieve the side effects of menstruation such as cramping and heavy bleeding. Raspberry leaf is said to strengthen the uterus in pregnant women. Yarrow is also a uterine tonic. White clover has analgesic properties, and lady's mantle offers antiaging properties and is known to ease menstrual pain, stop spotting between periods, and reduce a heavy flow.

Autumn Blend Tonic

Ingredients
• 4 tablespoons nettle • 3 tablespoons spearmint • 3 tablespoons lemon balm • 2 tablespoons mullein • 2 tablespoons dandelion leaf and root • 2 tablespoons red clover blossoms • 1 tablespoon rose hips
• 1 tablespoon dried ginger

Directions
• *Combine all of the dry ingredients and store in an airtight container such as a mason jar or tin.*
• *To brew, pour 1 cup of boiling water over 1½ teaspoons of the tea blend.*
• *Let it steep for 15 minutes to 8 hours. Then strain the herbs and enjoy hot or cold.*
• *Sweeten if desired with honey or a pinch of stevia.*

Benefits: Enjoy this herbal tonic each autumn to support your health as the cold winter months approach. Nettle eases muscle pain and boosts immunity and cardiovascular health, spearmint eases digestion and relieves stress, lemon balm elevates the spirits, mullein helps to battle infectious and inflammatory diseases such as colds and flu, dandelion supplies vitamins and acts as a diuretic, red clover helps regulate blood pressure and treats indigestion and respiratory issues, anti-inflammatory rose hips are loaded with vitamin C, and ginger eases stomach woes and can help reduce belly fat.

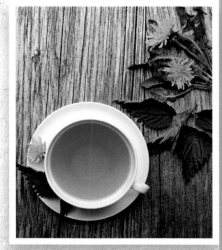

Autumn Blend Tonic

SLEEP-INDUCING TEAS

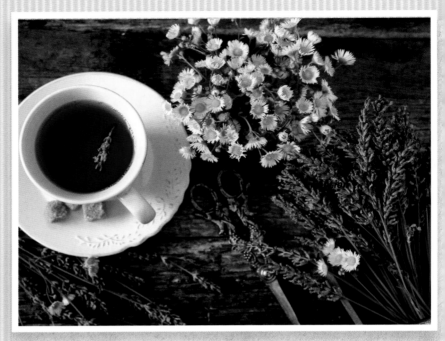

Sleepyhead Tea

Sleepyhead Tea

Ingredients

- 2 tablespoons chamomile
- 2 tablespoons dried lavender
- 1 tablespoon catnip
- 1 tablespoon peppermint
- Honey to taste

Directions

- *Combine herbs and place mixture in a container.*
- *Place a teaspoonful of the herbal mixture in a tea steeper or a small square of cheesecloth.*
- *Pour hot water over the top.*
- *Add honey if desired.*
- *Cover and let steep for 8 to 10 minutes.*

Benefits: This tea is loaded with calmatives that should send you off to dreamland in minutes. Chamomile and lavender are two of the best-regarded sleep-inducing herbs. Both mint and catnip, a variety of mint, have a calming effect on the stomach and the mind.

Sleep Tight Tea

Ingredients
- 2 tablespoons chamomile leaves
- 1 tablespoon hops flowers
- 1 tablespoon passionflower
- 1 tablespoon lemon balm
- 1 tablespoon peppermint leaf

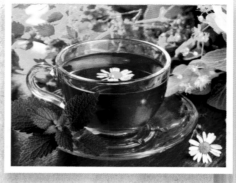

Sleep Tight Tea

Directions
- *Combine the herbs together in a bowl, then store in an airtight container when not in use. Label the blend and the date made.*
- *To prepare the tea, combine 1 to 2 tablespoons of the herb mixture with 1 to 1½ cups of boiling water.*
- *Allow to steep for 5 to 15 minutes before straining and drinking. The longer it steeps, the more potent it will be.*

Benefits: This tea is like a giant infusion of relaxation. The peppermint is added both for flavor and to help with indigestion, which can sometimes be a cause of sleeplessness. Chamomile and hops both calm the nerves. Lemon balm is prescribed for insomnia, while passionflower quiets the mind.

Sweet Dreams Tea

Ingredients
- 2 tablespoons spearmint
- 1 tablespoon chamomile
- 1 tablespoon Saint-John's-wort
- 1 tablespoon nettle leaf
- 1 tablespoon rosebuds
- 1 tablespoon dried orange or lemon peel

Directions
- *Mix the herbs together and place in a large infuser.*
- *Boil a quart of water. Pour the water into a large teapot and place the infuser inside it. Let the brew steep for 4 to 5 minutes.*
- *Sweeten with honey, if necessary.*

Benefits: This aromatic tea is the perfect aid to send you into a deep sleep. This is because all these herbs contribute different properties—some help with insomnia, others ease muscle aches, indigestion, tension, stress, and much more.

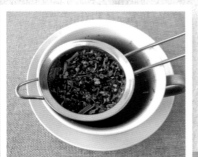

Sweet Dreams Tea

REFRESHING ICED TEAS

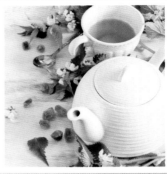

Nettle-Mint Summer Tea

Ingredients
- 1½ cups water
- 1 or 2 tablespoons of dried nettle
- 2 teaspoons peppermint or spearmint, dried or fresh

Nettle-Mint Summer Tea

Directions
- *Boil water and pour over loose herbs in a large mug.*
- *Let liquid steep for 20 minutes or up to a few hours.*
- *Strain and sweeten with honey or stevia, if desired.*
- *Transfer cooled tea to a tall glass and add ice.*
- *Garnish with mint leaves. Try adding a touch of cream, as well.*

Benefits: Iced teas provide the benefits of hot tea, but can be used in place of many high-calorie commercial soft drinks. In this recipe you can use either fresh or dried nettle, but the protein content in the dried leaves is higher than fresh, and you can't get fresh leaves all year round. Nettle is also full of vitamins, minerals, and amino acids. It acts as a tonic for female problems. Mint offers calming effects on the stomach and can help relieve depression.

Pink Lady Iced Tea

Ingredients
- 3 teaspoons green tea or two green tea bags
- 3 teaspoons chamomile
- ¼ cup hibiscus flowers
- 3 teaspoons orange peel
- 1 ounces dried raspberries, crushed a bit

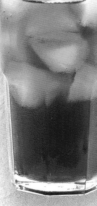

Directions
- *Blend the herbs and fruit together in a mason jar, cover, and shake to combine.*
- *Use approximately half the recipe to make a quart of iced tea. Pour boiling water over the tea mixture in a large saucepan, then cover and steep for 3 minutes at the most.*
- *Strain and pour into a pitcher with lots of ice.*
- *Use 1 heaping teaspoon to make 1 cup of hot tea.*

Pink Lady Iced Tea

Benefits: This refreshing pink tea makes a perfect midafternoon pick me up on a hot day. Green tea is a rich source of antioxidants and vital nutrients; chamomile induces calm; and hibiscus aids digestion, supports the immune system, and fights inflammation. Raspberries contain powerful antioxidants that combat cancer and heart disease and may be able to slow the aging process.

Lemon-Basil Iced Tea

Ingredients
- ½ lemon, thinly sliced
- 6 fresh basil leaves
- 2 green tea bags
- 3 cups hot water
- Raw honey, optional

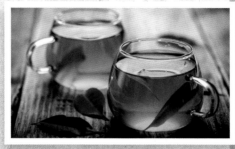

Lemon-Basil Iced Tea

Directions
- *Add the lemon slices, fresh basil leaves, and green tea bags to a 1-quart mason jar or pitcher.*
- *Pour hot water into the mason jar, and allow tea to steep for 15 minutes. Then remove the tea bags.*
- *Place in the fridge and chill for 3–4 hours to allow the flavors to release.*

Benefits: This tea provides thirst-quenching refreshment on a sultry summer afternoon. Plus it's packed with herbal goodness. Basil is an anti-inflammatory that benefits the digestion, fights depression, helps regulate blood sugar, and supports liver function. Green tea is loaded with antioxidants and nutrients.

Lime-Coconut Iced Tea

Ingredients
- 2 black tea bags
- ½ lime, thinly sliced
- 3 cups coconut water, heated
- Raw honey, optional

Lime-Coconut
Iced Tea

Directions
- *Add the black tea bags and sliced lime to a 1-quart mason jar or pitcher.*
- *Pour heated, but not boiling, coconut water into the mason jar and allow tea to steep for 15 minutes. Then remove the tea bags. Add honey to taste.*
- *Place in the refrigerator for 3 to 4 hours until it is chilled completely and the flavors have released.*

Benefits: This refreshing tea offers a little taste of the tropics along with its health benefits. Black tea contains antioxidants such as polyphenols that protect our cells from DNA damage, thus helping to combat cancer, heart disease, diabetes, and the ill effects of aging.

REFRESHING ICED TEAS

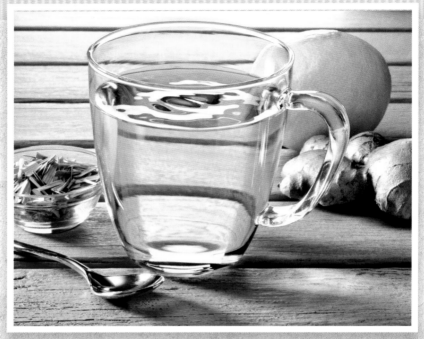

Peachy Ginger Tea

Peachy Ginger Tea

Ingredients
- 1 peach, pitted and sliced
- 2 green tea bags
- 1½ inches of fresh ginger, sliced into 4 rounds
- 3 cups hot water
- Raw honey, optional

Directions
- *Add the sliced peach and green tea bags to a 1-quart mason jar or pitcher.*
- *Skewer the sliced ginger rounds on a toothpick or wooden skewer to make them easier to remove, then add them to the jar.*
- *Pour the hot water into the mason jar, and allow to steep for 15 minutes. Then remove the tea bags. Add honey, if required.*
- *Place in the refrigerator for 3 to 4 hours until completely chilled and the flavors have released. Serve over ice.*

Benefits: This peachy tea has real Southern flair, plus peaches contain antioxidants and are rich in vitamins and minerals. The fresh ginger elevates the flavor as it supports digestion and helps burn fat. Green tea is brimming with cancer-fighting antioxidants and key nutrients.

Minty Blackberry Iced Tea

Ingredients
- ½ cup fresh blackberries
- 8 leaves fresh spearmint
- 2 bags green tea
- 3 cups hot water
- Raw honey, to taste

Directions
- *Add the fresh blackberries, mint leaves, and green tea bags to a large pitcher.*
- *Pour the hot water into the pitcher, and allow mixture to steep for 15 minutes. Then remove the tea bags. Add honey to taste.*
- *Place in the refrigerator until completely chilled, 3 to 4 hours.*

Benefits: This tasty tea offers both fruitful flavor and major health pluses. Blackberries provide impressive amounts of vitamin C as well as vitamin K, are high in manganese, and can help support brain health. Mint eases digestion and acts as a calmative; green tea is full of antioxidants that protect cells, and nutrients that also improve brain function.

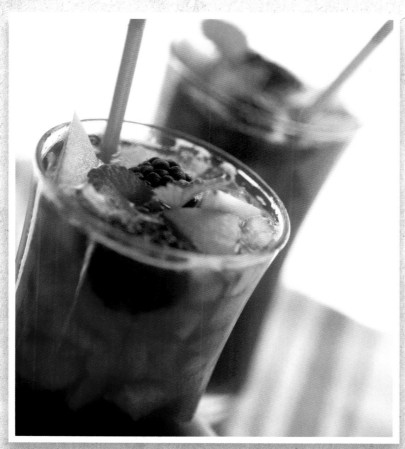

Minty Blackberry Iced Tea

HEALING TONICS

Herbal Spring Tonic

Ingredients
- 1 tablespoon heartsease
- 1 tablespoon nettle leaf
- 1½ cups water

Directions
- *Boil water.*
- *Mix in heartsease and nettle leaf, then steep for 15 minutes.*
- *Drink 3 times weekly for 2 weeks.*

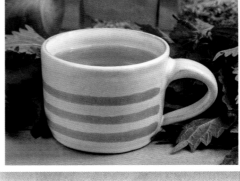

Herbal Spring Tonic

Benefits: Tonics are healing drinks meant to address specific issues and create a feeling of replenishment and vigor, especially after the hardships of winter. This recipe makes an excellent spring tonic drunk either hot or cold. Heartsease benefits the kidneys and the heart, and eases gout. It can also be blended with other teas. Nettle leaf is the premier spring tonic—a natural allergy remedy that benefits the skin, bones, and urinary tract.

Black Pepper Tonic

Ingredients
- 2 cups fresh water
- 1 teaspoon freshly ground black pepper
- 1 tablespoon honey
- 1 teaspoon lemon juice
- 1 heaping teaspoon grated ginger (optional)

Directions
- *Combine the water with the pepper, lemon juice, and grated ginger in a large mason jar.*
- *Mix well and then strain.*
- *Add the honey, mix again, and drink neat or over ice.*

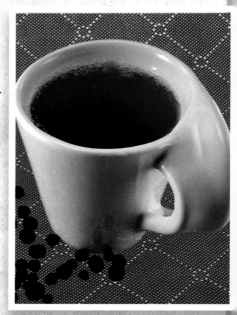

Black Pepper Tonic

Benefits: This invigorating tonic is the perfect way to combat fatigue and soothe anxiety. The black pepper is full of antioxidants, the honey is a natural antiseptic, and the ginger supports the stomach and intestines and helps to clear out respiratory passages.

Lavender-Lemon Tonic

Ingredients
- 4 cups water
- ¼ cup fresh crushed lavender flowers
- ¾ cup fresh lemon juice, or to taste
- ¾ cup honey, or to taste

Directions
- *Bring 2 cups of water to a boil, remove from heat, and stir in honey.*
- *Add lavender, cover, and steep for 20 minutes or a half hour.*
- *Strain the beverage,* pour into a pitcher, and stir in the lemon juice.
- *Add final 2 cups of water, stir, and place in refrigerator to chill.*

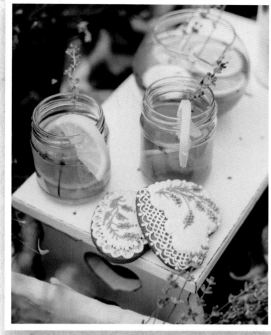

Lavender-Lemon Tonic

Benefits: Lavender-lemon tonic is tart and refreshing. Lavender contains powerful antioxidants to boost the immune system as well as offering mentally calming effects. Lemon juice furnishes vitamin C and has healthful astringent properties.

Lemon Turmeric Flush Tonic

Ingredients
- 2 cups water
- 1 lemon, squeezed
- ½ teaspoon ground turmeric
- ¼ teaspoon ground ginger
- ⅛ teaspoon cayenne pepper (optional)
- ⅛ teaspoon cinnamon
- 1½ teaspoon stevia, honey, or real maple syrup

Directions
- *Mix together water, lemon juice, turmeric, ginger, cayenne pepper, and cinnamon.*
- *Add stevia, honey, or maple syrup to taste.*
- *The optional cayenne pepper adds a kick to the mixture, but not everyone can handle it. Serves 2*

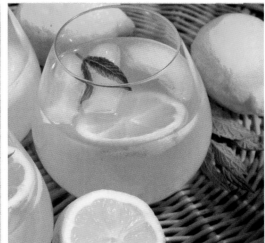

Lemon Turmeric Flush Tonic

HEALING TONICS

Benefits: This is a great detoxifying tonic that can help your body rid itself of toxin and pollutants.

Turmeric-Milk Tonic for Sore Throat

Ingredients
- ½ tsp dried turmeric powder
- 1 tsp fresh ginger, minced
- ¼ cup water
- ¾ cup milk

Directions
- *Blend liquid and dry ingredients and heat the mixture for a few minutes, until the milk almost boils.*
- *If you want to add ¼ teaspoon of peppercorns, which are thought to improve the absorption of the turmeric, do so before heating. For extra flavor try adding a few pods of cardamom (cracked) and a pinch of saffron to the liquid before heating.*
- *Let the mixture cool slightly, then strain and drink.*

Benefits: This traditional tonic for sore or raspy throats will help ease pain and reduce inflammation. Turmeric is a natural anti-inflammatory and painkiller that inhibits COX-2, which is an enzyme that speeds up the production of chemical messengers called prostaglandins that promote inflammation. As a result, turmeric has been used for many centuries in Chinese medicine to treat arthritis and rheumatism. Fresh ginger is an anti-inflammatory that reduces pain and soreness as well as supporting digestion.

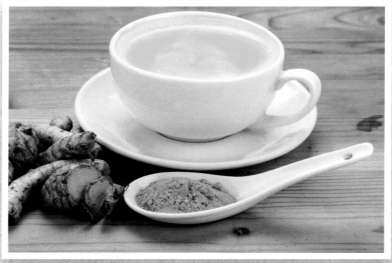

Turmeric-Milk Tonic

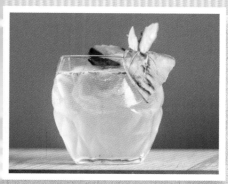

Basil-Birch Urinary Aid Tonic

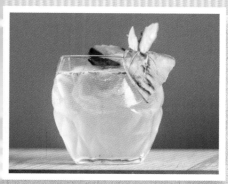

Basil-Birch Urinary Aid Tonic

Basil-Birch Urinary Aid Tonic

Ingredients
- 2 teaspoons fresh basil
- 2 teaspoons birch leaves
- 1 cup water

Directions
- *Boil the water and pour it into a mug over the basil and birch leaves.*
- *Steep for 10 minutes, then strain.*
- *Drink 1 cup 3 times daily until urinary symptoms are gone.*

Benefits: Basil is effective for use against bladder or kidney inflammation. Birch leaves are great sources of vitamin C and are a long-respected treatment for urinary infections. They also act as a diuretic that increases urinary output, thus removing toxins from the body and speeding up the healing process.

Fresh Sorrel Juice Tonic

Ingredients
- 2 lbs. carrots, cleaned
- 2 stalks celery, washed
- 1 apple, cored and divided into eighths
- ½ to 1 bunch sorrel

Directions
- *Run 2 carrots through juicer or blender.*
- *Add celery and sorrel, then alternate carrots and apple slices.*
- *Strain through cheesecloth and drink chilled.*

Benefits: Try this healthy, detoxifying tonic, which is packed with vitamins and minerals and the antioxidant benefits of fruits and vegetables. Carrots provide vitamin A, antioxidants, and fiber. Celery is a storehouse of vitamins B6, C, and K, as well as potassium. Sorrel is known as a diuretic that helps to regulate blood pressure, lower cholesterol, and improve circulation; it also boosts the immune system.

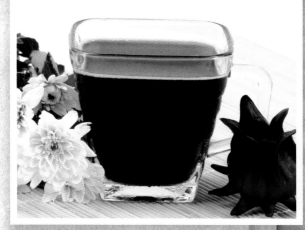

Fresh Sorrel Juice Tonic

AYURVEDIC TONICS

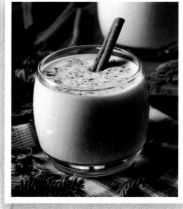

Ojas-building Tonic

Ingredients
- 1 tablespoon chopped dates
- 2 teaspoons chopped almonds
- 1 tablespoon coconut meat or flakes
- ½ teaspoon saffron
- 1 or 2 teaspoons ghee
- ⅛ teaspoon green cardamom
- 1 cup almond milk
- 1 teaspoon raw honey

Ojas-building Tonic

- ⅛ teaspoon or one 500mg capsule of ojas-building herbs: shatavari ("strength of 100 husbands") or ashwagandha ("strength of ten horses").

Directions
- *Add small amounts of the first 6 ingredients to one cup of milk as you slowly bring it to a boil.*
- *Add ojas-building herbs to the milk.*
- *Once the milk, herbs, and spices are heated and off the burner, add 1 teaspoon of raw honey.*
- *Drink one cup each night for 3 months to rebuild ojas levels and support sleep patterns.*

Benefits: Ayurvedic medicine is a large part of the ancient healing traditions of India. By following ayurvedic guidelines for eating, you will feel nourished and energized. According to ayurvedic writings, stress depletes a precious substance in the body called ojas, the physiological expression of consciousness, in charge of immunity, reproduction, beauty, and overall health. Ojas takes 30 days to be manufactured in the body. The blend of fruits and spices in this tonic will put you well on your way to rebuilding your ojas.

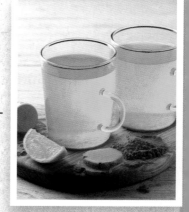

Lemon-Turmeric Tonic

Ingredients
- 1 teaspoon raw honey
- 1 teaspoon fresh squeezed lemon
- 1 teaspoon turmeric
- ¼ teaspoon cayenne pepper

Lemon-Turmeric Tonic

Directions

- Place the honey in a mug or cup.
- Squeeze a teaspoon or so of fresh lemon juice over the honey and mix. The honey will dissolve into the lemon juice.
- Add your turmeric and your cayenne pepper.
- Mix thoroughly and enjoy lemon-turmeric tonic.
- Another option is to combine the tonic with a cup of your favorite fruit juice or herbal tea.

Benefits: Curcumin, turmeric's main active ingredient, has the power to fight two devastating ailments: heart disease and cancer. The spice, with its powerful anti-inflammatory and antioxidant properties, has also been effective in treating and preventing arthritis and depression. Cayenne pepper is antifungal, antibacterial, anti-inflammatory, stimulates digestion and circulation, thins blood clots, and has cancer-fighting properties. Lemons are full of antioxidants, potassium, and vitamin C. Fresh-squeezed lemon juice boosts digestive enzymes and promotes a healthy pH balance.

Basic Turmeric-Milk Tonic

Ingredients

- ½ inch of fresh ginger, grated
- ½ teaspoon dried turmeric powder or 1-inch piece of fresh turmeric
- 1 cup whole milk
- ½ cup spring water
- 1 tablespoon raw honey, or to taste

Directions

- Place all the ingredients except honey into a pan and simmer for 20 minutes.
- Let sit for 15 minutes to steep.
- Rewarm if needed and then add the honey.
- Once the honey has been stirred in, strain and drink.

Benefits: Turmeric's main active ingredient has been shown to combat two serious ailments: heart disease and cancer. The spice has powerful anti-inflammatory and antioxidant properties that have also been effective in treating and preventing arthritis and depression. Ginger can soothe indigestion and offer pain-relieving analgesic effects.

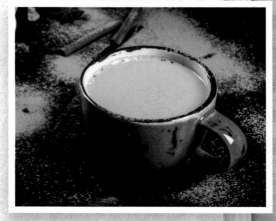

Basic Turmeric-Milk Tonic

AYURVEDIC TONICS

Sour Apple–Kale Tonic

Ingredients
- 1 whole apple, cored
- 1 inch fresh ginger, grated
- 1 pound kale, shredded
- ½ whole lemon
- 1 cup spring water
- honey, to taste

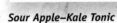
Sour Apple–Kale Tonic

Directions
- *Squeeze the juice from the lemon and cut up the apple and place in blender.*
- *Make sure the kale is chopped fairly fine before you add it, or you may need to toss it in a food processor before blending.*
- *Add ginger and water and process until smooth. then strain, and drink.*

Benefits: This tonic makes a great wake-up beverage, tart, sweet, and full of vitamins. Apples are rich in antioxidants and fiber, and their phytonutrients may even reduce the risk of cancer, diabetes, and heart disease. Kale is a source of many vitamins and minerals, especially K, C, A, and B vitamins; it is high in fiber and water and detoxifies the liver by stimulating the release of bile. Lemon brings its astringent properties as well as vitamin C and potassium.

Anti-Bloat Spice Tonic

Ingredients
- 2 cups spring water
- ¼ teaspoon cumin seeds
- ¼ teaspoon coriander seeds
- ¼ teaspoon fennel seeds

Directions
- *Set the water to boil.*
- *Toast the seeds in a small, dry frying pan over medium heat, until they become aromatic.*
- *Transfer the seeds to a mortar and pestle—you can*

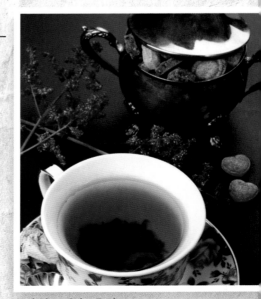
Anti-Bloat Spice Tonic

also use a cutting board and the side of a cleaver—and bruise them slightly.

• Place the seeds to steep in the boiled water for 5 minutes or until the mixture cools to a comfortable drinking temperature.

• Strain out the spices, and serve. Makes 2 servings.

Benefits: This ayurvedic tonic is effective for detoxification, digestion, and reducing uncomfortable bloating and gas. It stimulates the metabolism and clears out excess water, simultaneously cleansing the urinary tract and reducing inflammation. The mildly bitter carminative seeds amp up the detoxification process, purify the blood, and help to soothe tension. Toasting the seeds releases their volatile organic compounds, increasing both their flavor and health benefits.

Grape Juice–Cardamom Tonic

Ingredients
• 2 pinches ground green cardamom (or open pods and crush seeds with a mortar and pestle)
• ¼ inch fresh ginger
• 1 cup organic grape juice
• 2 pinches turmeric

Directions
• Mash fresh ginger with a mortar and pestle or the side of a cleaver.
• Mix ginger, organic grape juice, and the other spices together in a glass. For best results let

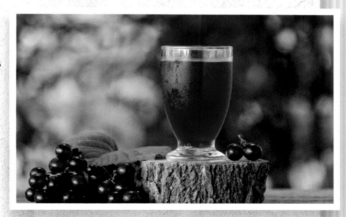

Grape Juice–Cardamom Tonic

mixture steep for 20 minutes at room temperature.
• Add ⅛ teaspoon of the herb ashwagandha for a more powerful toning and rejuvenating effect.

Benefits: Try this sweet, refreshing tonic if you are feeling sluggish or bloated. Grapes are one of the chosen fruits in ayurvedic medicine. They are believed to nourish blood plasma, cool the blood, and refresh and rejuvenate the spirit. They have a gentle laxative effect and are slightly astringent. Turmeric invigorates and cleanses the blood. Cardamom and ginger both aid in digestion, clearing the stomach to create a feeling of lightness.

INDIAN AND MIDDLE EASTERN BEVERAGES

Mango Lassi

Ingredients
- 1 cup plain yogurt
- ½ cup milk
- 1 cup chopped ripe mango, frozen chopped mango, or a cup of canned mango pulp
- 4 teaspoons honey or sugar, to taste
- A dash of ground green cardamom, or open pods and crush seeds with mortar and pestle
- Ice

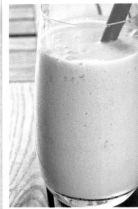

Mango Lassi

Directions
- *Put the mango, yogurt, milk, sugar, and cardamom into a blender and blend for 2 minutes.*
- *If you want a more milkshake-like consistency, blend in some ice. If you want the drink colder, serve over ice cubes.*
- *Sprinkle with a tiny pinch of ground cardamom to serve. The lassi can be kept refrigerated for up to 24 hours.*

Benefits: This is a customer favorite in Indian restaurants all over the world. Yogurt provides calcium and active yeast cultures. Mango is known to have antioxidant compounds that protect against certain forms of cancer; the fruit also lowers cholesterol, clears the skin, improves eye health, aids digestion, and may help regulate blood sugar. Depending on how ripe and sweet the mango is—or if you are using canned, sweetened mango pulp—you will need to add more or less sweetener to the lassi.

Persian Pomegranate Cooler

Ingredients
- 16 ounces pomegranate juice
- 4 ounces fresh squeezed lemon juice
- 1 teaspoon orange blossom water
- ¼ cup sugar (or more, to taste)
- 20 ounces club soda or 20 ounces sparkling water

Directions
- *Mix the pomegranate juice, lemon juice, orange*

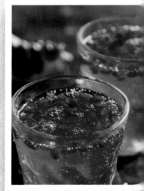

Persian Pomegranate Cooler

blossom water, and sugar until the sugar dissolves.
- Pour 5 ounces of the mixture into a tall glass and slowly add 5 ounces of club soda, stirring slowly.
- Add several ice cubes to chill, and serve.

Benefits: This refreshing drink is enjoyed throughout Iran and other parts of the Middle East. Pomegranate juice is full of antioxidants and anti-inflammatories and may be a factor in preventing cancer, heart disease, arthritis, and Alzheimer's disease. Orange blossom water or orange flower water is a clear, aromatic byproduct of the distillation of bitter orange blossoms for their essential oils. It is widely used in aromatherapy, cosmetics, and cooking. It softens the skin, eases stomach distress, and calms the nerves.

Limonana

Ingredients
- 6 tablespoons sugar
- ½ cup plus 6 tablespoons water, divided
- ½ cup fresh lemon juice
- 1–2 drops orange blossom water
- 4–6 stems worth of mint leaves (about 30 or 40 leaves) with the stems discarded, plus a few extra sprigs for garnish, if desired
- 15 ice cubes

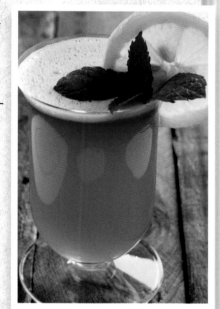

Limonana

Directions
- Add the sugar and 6 tablespoons of water to a small saucepan.
- Heat over medium heat, stirring constantly, until the sugar is dissolved.
- Cool to room temperature.
- Add the cooled sugar syrup, remaining ½ cup water, lemon juice, mint leaves, ice cubes, and orange blossom water to a blender.
- Pulse a few times to break up the ice and then process until slushy.
- Pour into 2 tall glasses, garnish with mint leaves if desired, and serve immediately. Makes 2 servings.

Benefits: This frozen lemonade with mint is popular in the Middle East, where sipping cool beverages is a way of life. Because the recipe adds ice, the lemonade should be fairly concentrated to begin with. Mint is a flavor enhancer and digestive aid that contains antioxidants. Orange blossom water or orange flower water is a clear, aromatic byproduct of the distillation of bitter orange blossoms for their essential oils. It is similar to rose water, another frequent addition to Middle Eastern and Mediterranean cuisine.

LATIN AMERICAN BEVERAGES

Yerba Mate

Ingredients
- 1 cup spring water
- 1 tablespoon yerba mate

Directions
- *Wet the yerba mate leaves slightly with cold water, then pour hot, not boiling, water over them.*
- *Steep for 5 minutes, strain, and serve.*
- *Traditionally this drink is served in hollowed-out gourds with silver rims.*

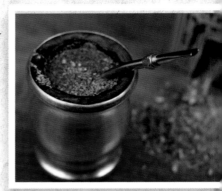

Yerba Mate

Benefits: The benefits of this South American favorite are similar to those of green tea. Its high antioxidant levels reduce oxidative stress. It also provides substantial amounts of minerals and vitamins such as potassium, manganese, phosphorus, sodium, and nitrogen, and vitamins A, C, and E. It promotes a healthy digestive tract and cardiovascular system and improves digestion. Flavor-wise, the sticks and stems will typically supply more of a woodsy taste than pure leaf mate will. As with other bitter beverages such as black coffee, beer, or tea, drinking straight yerba mate may be an acquired taste.

Mexican Hot Chocolate

Ingredients
- 2 cups water
- 2 cups milk
- 5¼ ounces quality dark chocolate (75% cacao or more), coarsely chopped
- ½ to 1 teaspoon cinnamon powder
- ⅓ cup granulated sugar, or to taste
- Pinch cayenne pepper
- Cocoa powder, for garnish
- 4 cinnamon sticks, for garnish

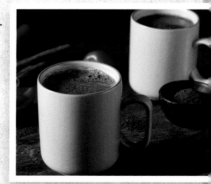

Mexican Hot Chocolate

Directions
- *Pour the milk and water into a saucepan and bring to a boil.*
- *When the milk and water mixture is boiling, take it off the stove and add the chocolate, mixing vigorously with a whisk.*

- Add cinnamon and cayenne, and stir. Add sugar to taste.
- Garnish with a cinnamon stick and serve with a dusting of cocoa powder. Makes 4 cups.

Benefits: This hot chocolate is based on a real Mexican recipe and incorporates dark chocolate, which is now known to provide heart-healthy benefits. Plus, the ingredients in this recipe are real foods, not the many additives and preservatives you'll find in commercial hot cocoa packets. You can play around with this recipe—and amp up its nutrient value—by adding other spices, such as nutmeg, cloves, allspice, or vanilla beans.

Coquito

Ingredients
- 1 15-oz. can cream of coconut
- 1 14-oz. can sweetened condensed milk
- 1 13.5-oz. can coconut milk
- 2 12-oz. cans evaporated milk
- ¾ cup white rum (optional)
- 1 teaspoon vanilla extract
- ½ teaspoon ground cinnamon
- ¼ teaspoon ground cloves
- ¼ teaspoon ground nutmeg, plus more for garnish

Directions
- Process cream of coconut, sweetened condensed milk, and coconut milk in a blender or food processor until completely smooth. Transfer mixture to a large bowl or pitcher.
- Whisk in the evaporated milk, rum, vanilla, ground cinnamon, and nutmeg.
- Cover and chill for 24 hours.
- Garnish with nutmeg and cinnamon sticks, if desired. Serving size: ½ cup.

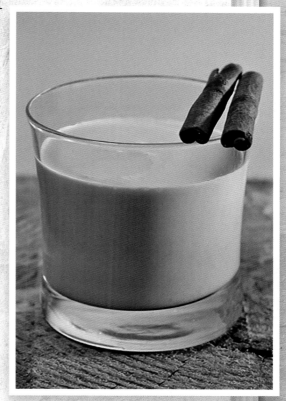

Coquito

Benefits: For many Puerto Ricans—and other Latinos—it's not Christmas without coquito. This drink, like many holiday beverages, is rather high in calories, but it does contain beneficial spices such as nutmeg, cloves, and cinnamon. Because it's very rich, it can be served over ice if you want to dilute it. A typical Christmas coquito includes rum, but this alcohol-free version is favored by children and adults alike. Other fruit flavors, such as guava or pineapple, can be added to the recipe.

NUTRITIOUS BREAKFAST SMOOTHIES

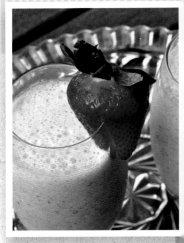

Fruit Basket Smoothie

Ingredients
- 1 cup fresh or frozen strawberries
- ½ cup crushed, cubed, or sliced pineapple
- 1 banana
- 2 cups orange juice
- ½ cup Greek yogurt
- 1 cup baby spinach
- 1 tablespoon chia or flax seeds
- Ice

Fruit Basket Smoothie

Directions
- *Combine ingredients in a blender and blend until smooth and creamy.*
- *Add ice depending on how chilled you want the smoothie.*
Note: Frozen bananas work best in smoothies. Peel, slice in half, place banana in a large zip-seal bag, and leave in the freezer overnight.

Benefits: Start your day with a healthy blend of your favorite fruits. Strawberries are full of fiber and contain high levels of antioxidants. They make ideal snack foods—low calorie, cholesterol free, fat free, and sodium free. They are also good sources of manganese and potassium. Bananas are rich in nutrients, and pineapples provide the enzyme bromelian, which is an anti-inflammatory that promotes digestive health. Orange juice is a good source of vitamin C, and spinach has an overall high nutrient value.

Tropical Sunrise Spiced Smoothie

Ingredients
- 1 cup fresh or canned peaches
- 1 cup fresh or canned mango
- 1 banana
- 1 cup fresh, frozen, or carton orange juice
- ¼ teaspoon turmeric
- ¼ teaspoon ground ginger

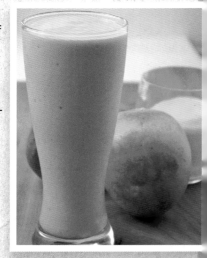

Tropical Sunrise Spiced Smoothie

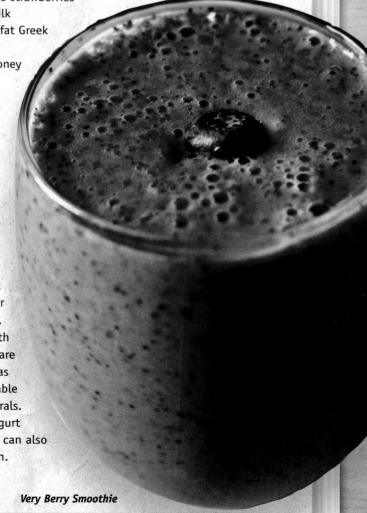

Directions

• Add ingredients into a blender and blend until smooth and creamy.
• Add ice, depending on how cold you like your smoothies.
Note: Frozen bananas work best in smoothies. Peel, slice in half, place in a large zip-seal bag, and leave in the freezer overnight.

Benefits: This delicious smoothie makes an ideal breakfast on those busy days when you need to be out the door in a flash. The peaches and mangoes are a good source of vitamin C as well as other micronutrients, and the orange juice is also rich in vitamin C. The banana offers a healthy mix of vitamins and minerals, including essential potassium.

Very Berry Smoothie

Ingredients

• 1½ medium bananas, peeled and frozen
• ½ cup frozen raspberries
• ½ cup fresh or frozen blueberries
• 1 cup fresh whole strawberries
• ½ cup nonfat milk
• ¼ cup plain nonfat Greek yogurt
• 2 tablespoons honey

Directions

• Place ingredients in blender; blend until smooth.
• Pour into a tall glass and garnish with a berry or two.

Benefits: This smoothie maxes out on antioxidant berries, which offer vitamins, minerals, and a host of health benefits. Bananas are rich in potassium as well as other valuable vitamins and minerals. Probiotic Greek yogurt offers calcium and can also help with digestion.

Very Berry Smoothie

THERAPEUTIC SMOOTHIES

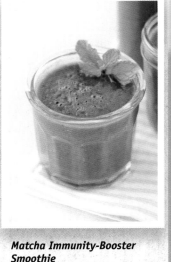

Matcha Immunity-Booster Smoothie

Ingredients
- 1 small or half large banana, frozen
- 2 teaspoons pure matcha powder OR 1 scoop green tea latte powder
- 1 mandarin orange, peeled
- ⅓ cup vanilla Greek yogurt
- ⅓ cup milk of choice (cow's, almond, soy, etc.)
- 1 scoop unflavored protein powder

Matcha Immunity-Booster Smoothie

Directions
- *Place all ingredients into blender and blend on high until smooth and desired consistency is achieved.*
- *For added nutrition, consider adding 1–3 teaspoons of flax, chia, or hemp seeds.*
- *Serve in a tall glass garnished with orange peel.*

Benefits: Antioxidant matcha powder is full of flavor—it also boosts the metabolism, calms the mind, and relaxes the body. It's rich in chlorophyll, fiber, and vitamins. Bananas are a good source of essential vitamins and minerals. The mandarin orange supplies vitamin C and fiber. Greek yogurt provides probiotics, and its acidity enables the body to absorb nutrients more easily.

Purple Pick-Me-Up Smoothie

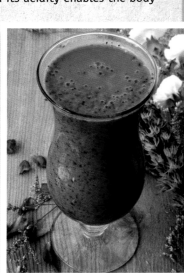

Ingredients
- ½ cup frozen cherries
- ½ cup frozen or fresh blueberries
- ½ cup frozen sliced peaches or mangoes
- 1 cup packed spring mix salad greens
- 1 cup milk or unsweetened almond or cashew milk
- 1 cup plain yogurt or plain Greek yogurt
- 1 tsp vanilla extract

Directions
- *Add all the ingredients to a blender, and process until creamy.*

Purple Pick-Me-Up Smoothie

- *Pour into a tall glass and garnish the rim with a few berries.*

Note: For best consistency and easiest blending with Bullet-style blenders, try putting fruit, yogurt, or protein first, doing a quick blend, then adding greens and milk or liquid.

Benefits: This smoothie is ideal for replenishing your system after strenuous workouts at the gym. The cherries and blueberries provide antioxidants that keep inflammation down and promote recovery after exercise. Sweet cherries contain anthocyanins and quercetin that may help combat cancer. If you use tart cherries, you may have more restful sleep due to the melatonin they provide. Peaches and mangoes provide fiber and antioxidant vitamin C as well as many other essential micronutrients.

Berry Belly-Fat-Blaster Smoothie

Ingredients
- 1 cup plain low-fat Greek yogurt
- 1 cup frozen berries (blueberries, strawberries, or açai berries are all good choices)
- 1 tablespoon vanilla extract
- 1 tablespoon chia seeds
- ½ cup ice

Directions
- *In a blender, combine the yogurt, berries, vanilla, ground chia seeds, and ice.*
- *Blend on high for 1 minute, or until desired consistency is reached. Serve cold. Makes 1 serving.*

Benefits: This delicious berry smoothie can help you shed that stubborn "muffin top"—it provides high levels of omega-3 fatty acids, which help to reduce stress hormones that pack on stubborn belly fat. The Greek yogurt provides a quality source of protein to help you feel full. Berries contain antioxidants and are high in fiber—strawberries may help preserve memory as we age; blueberries contribute to heart health and lower cholesterol; and raspberries contain a compound called ellagic acid that exhibits anti-cancer properties.

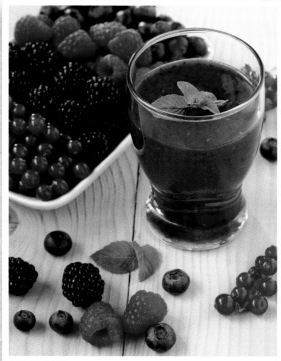

Berry Belly-Fat-Blaster Smoothie

INDEX

INDEX

INDEX

PICTURE CREDITS